PATIENT MANAGEMENT PROBLEMS IN PSYCHIATRY

D0531157

For Churchill Livingstone:

Publisher: Georgina Bentliff
Editorial Co-ordination: Editorial Resources Unit
Production Controller: Nancy Henry
Design: Design Resources Unit
Sales Promotion Executive: Hilary Brown

9.95

CEFN COED HOSPITAL
MEDICAL LIBRARY

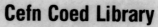

Cefn Coed Library

Z000566

WITHDRAWN 05/05/24
RM.

PATIENT MANAGEMENT PROBLEMS IN PSYCHIATRY

FOR THE MRCPsych ORAL EXAMINATION

Parimala Moodley MBChB MRCPsych
Senior Lecturer, Community Mental Health
Institute of Psychiatry, London

Rajini Ramana MBBS MRCPsych
Senior Registrar, The Maudsley and
the Bethlem Royal Hospitals, London

Luiz Dratcu MD MSc MRCPsych
Honorary Senior Registrar, The Maudsley and
the Bethlem Royal Hospitals, London

Foreword by
R.H. Cawley PhD BSc MBChB FRCPscyh FRCP (Lond) DPMEng
Emeritus Professor of Psychological Medicine,
University of London, London

CHURCHILL LIVINGSTONE
EDINBURGH LONDON MELBOURNE NEW YORK AND TOKYO 1991

CHURCHILL LIVINGSTONE
Medical Division of Longman Group UK Limited

Distributed in the United States of America by
Churchill Livingstone Inc., 1560 Broadway, New
York, N.Y. 10036, and by associated companies,
branches and representatives throughout the
world.

© Longman Group UK Limited 1991

All rights reserved. No part of this publication may
be reproduced, stored in a retrieval system, or
transmitted in any form or by any means,
electronic, mechanical, photocopying, recording
or otherwise, without either the prior written
permission of the publishers (Churchill
Livingstone, Robert Stevenson House,
1–3 Baxter's Place, Leith Walk, Edinburgh EH1
3AF), or a licence permitting restricted copying in
the United Kingdom issued by the Copyright
Licensing Agency Ltd, 90 Tottenham Court Road,
WIP 9HE.

First published 1991

ISBN 0-443-04374-4

British Library Cataloguing in Publication Data
A catalogue record for this book is available from the British Library.

Produced by Longman Singapore Publisher (Pte) Ltd
Printed in Singapore

Foreword

Accurate clinical reasoning is at the heart of competent medical practice. A skill often neglected, it consists of attending closely to the specific problems of the individual patient, and applying knowledge, experience and imagination to analysing the predicament and its context, thus reaching a balanced appraisal of what actions are called for. Clinical reasoning is the basis of decisions regarding clinical management, which comprises the interacting processes of assessment and treatment.

Each specialty has its own needs and styles in its clinical reasoning. Management problems in psychiatry arise from a confluence of biomedical, psychosocial and personal themes applied to individual situations. Reasoning which does less than justice to each of these classes of variables is liable to be incorrect, even dangerous. That is why it has been found necessary to test the power and accuracy of the MRCPsych candidate's clinical reasoning not only in the clinical examination itself but also in the Patient Management Problems (PMP) Oral.

The prospective candidate is wise to reflect on precisely how the questions may be framed, and on the range covered by the test. As with all examinations, opportunity to rehearse is invaluable. Dr Moodley and her colleagues offer guidance together with a set of PMPs covering a wide field of clinical psychiatry. Their book can be recommended for preparing both for the examination and for the enhanced responsibilities which will follow success. It is a useful addition to the literature of basic postgraduate psychiatry.

R.H.C.

Preface

The Royal College of Psychiatrists introduced the new Patient Management Problem (PMP) Oral Examination in April 1988. Prior to this, the standards in the oral part of the MRCPsych Examination were demonstrably uneven and the new format sought to standardise this part of the examination.

The format of the examination is unique in that the candidate has to present the examiners with the practical assessment and management of the problem given, on the basis of a brief outline. Over the last 2 years, we have spoken to candidates taking the examination and have analysed the types of questions asked. We have also been helping candidates prepare for the examination by holding practice sessions, and this experience showed us that candidates need to be especially prepared for the PMP examination. Most candidates are uncertain about what to expect and find it difficult to answer the questions concisely. On the basis of our enquiries, we felt there was a need for a book specifically aimed at this part of the examination and decided to take on the task ourselves.

All fields of clinically relevant activity are covered. Some topics have been covered in much greater detail, especially where it is difficult to find adequate information in current standard textbooks. However, this book is not meant to cover all aspects of clinical management in psychiatry: it is an aid to preparation for the PMP Oral Examination.

We are most grateful to Dr Vishwajit Nimgaonkar, Dr Ann Gath, and Dr Ashok Venkitaraman for their comments on the first draft. We are particularly grateful to Dr Robin Jacoby and Professor R. H. Cawley for their invaluable help in the preparation of this book. We wish also to thank Lillian Gaywood for her help in the preparation of the manuscript.

We hope candidates will find this book useful as an aid in the preparation for their examinations.

1991
Parimala Moodley
Rajini Ramana
Luiz Dratcu

Guidelines to using this book

The PMP Oral Examination is a test of the candidate's ability to apply theoretical knowledge, practical experience and judgement to individual clinical situations of the kind one is likely to meet in future work. In the half hour devoted to this part of the examination the candidate will be presented with three or more distinct management problems. The questions are focused on practical management including accurate assessment of the patient and the problem. Candidates are required to impress upon the examiners that they have grasped the particular features of the case and that their clinical reasoning is sound. They are not required to produce a long disquisition. All the information given by the examiners has some clinical relevance. Sociodemographic details are clues to the individual features of the case, as are life events or situations. It is useful therefore to have a diagnostic formulation in mind in order to tackle the answer in a systematic manner. There should always be an attempt to start with the broad view before concentrating on specific details. It may be useful to summarise the main problems raised by the question quickly before starting the answer. This helps to organise one's thoughts and lets the examiners know that one has grasped the essence of the problem.

As the candidate goes along, the examiners may give further information that may alter the candidate's opinion about management. If the candidate thinks any additional information is needed in the course of his answer, it is best to ask the examiners. One should aim to convince the examiners that all aspects of the assessment and management of the case have been considered. If you are particularly confident of any one aspect, try to lead the examiner to this, subtly. Similarly, if one is not confident about any particular aspect, one should try to lead them around it without letting one's ignorance show.

Although the examination concentrates on the management of clinical problems, it is not unusual for candidates to be asked to give the differential diagnosis of a particular condition. There is also the expectation that candidates will be aware of recent advances in a given field.

In this book, questions have been arranged such that any consecutive four could represent what would be asked in the course of the 30 minutes. Some topics such as self-injurious behaviour have been covered in greater detail, as it is difficult to find adequate information on these topics in standard textbooks. Some questions are accompanied by a flow diagram that should help the candidate to practise a logical approach. Candidates are advised to rehearse the questions with colleagues and to formulate their answers before reading those in the book.

Some questions have a number of different elements to them, e.g. a young mother of three, whose husband has been posted abroad, complains of having difficulty coping and is feeling depressed because her eldest son, aged 5, who has just started school, has become enuretic. The examiners may want the candidate to talk about depression in a young women with three children under the age of 5, who has no close confidante, or they may want one to talk about management of enuresis, or both. In the book, we have concentrated on one of these issues for ease of presentation.

We have included references of particular importance and those that are relevant to individual questions. Standard textbooks have not been referenced, as it is assumed that at this stage the candidates have a broad base of psychiatric knowledge. A list of standard texts has been included at the end of the book.

Contents

Questions

Q1

A 30-year-old brewery worker is referred to you by his general practitioner. For the last 6 months he has become increasingly suspicious about his wife and is convinced she is having an affair. His wife went to the general practitioner, at her wits' end, saying she was fed up with the way he was continually looking for evidence of her infidelity and that she had felt quite scared of him on occasions. What is the problem and how would you deal with it?

Q2

A 13-year-old girl in school appears 'severely depressed'. The social worker rings you at 3 p.m. on Friday afternoon to ask for advice. How would you deal with it?

Q3

A 70-year-old widow comes to your outpatients' clinic. She has been receiving lorazepam 1 mg b.d. since her husband died 15 years ago. She now wants to come off the drug because she saw a TV programme where they said it was 'poisonous'. She is 'extremely worried' and still has trouble sleeping. Years ago, she was admitted to a psychiatric hospital and was treated with electroconvulsive therapy for her depression. How would you deal with this case?

Q4

A solicitor telephones you and requests you to see his client, a 58-year-old banker who was arrested for indecent exposure, with a view to writing a court report. He requests you to see him in your next outpatient clinic, which is the next day, as his client is now on bail, awaiting trial. What would you do?

Q5

You are called to the accident and emergency department to see a 24-year-old girl who weighs 38 kg (6 st). Her mother says that she had had 'anorexia' in the past. The patient was married, but separated a year ago and is now living with her mother, who has attended with the patient, and her mother's current boyfriend. How would you manage this?

Q6

A male colleague speaks to you 'in confidence' to tell you that he has been having an affair, unknown to his wife. His ex-general practitioner, who is also a friend, has just told him that his girlfriend is human immunodeficiency virus (HIV)-antibody-positive. He asks you if he should have a test and is quite worried about the possible outcome. How would you counsel him? He also tells you that even if he is HIV-antibody-positive, he will not tell his wife and forbids you to do so. Will you tell his wife? What are your legal responsibilities?

Q7

A.   A 6-year-old boy is brought by his parents to your outpatients' clinic. He has been wetting his bed since he was taken out of nappies, 2 years ago. How would you manage him?
B.   Bell and pad method proved successful, but the boy started bedwetting again after 1 month of continence. How would you proceed?

Q8

A general practitioner calls you to see a 65-year-old man, living alone, with auditory hallucinations and odd behaviour. He has not had any similar problems before.
A.   What would be your thoughts about the causes on your way to the patient's house?
B.   On assessment you find that he appears to have impaired hearing. What would you do?

Q9

A 6-year-old boy who is mentally retarded is brought to you by his mother. For the last 6 months, he has been banging his head, and pinching and scratching himself repeatedly and his arms and legs are covered with scars and recent injuries. The mother has been unable to get him to stop his behaviour. It has resulted in her having to spend more time with her son, which she finds difficult as she has recently divorced and needs to work full-time. How will you manage this problem?

Q10

A 58-year-old man who has been a day patient at your hospital has not been seen for 3 days. Prior to this, the staff felt that he was looking rather withdrawn and sad. He has a long history of depression. He lives on his own. How would you deal with this?

Q11

The casualty medical officer calls you to see a young and rather frail man who was admitted overnight. He was brought to the accident and emergency department by his friends after having two fainting episodes. He became extremely disturbed and agitated while he was being examined, and drew blood from a staff member after biting him. The staff are concerned about this, as they have noticed needle marks. He has been sedated for the time-being with chlorpromazine, to which he responded very quickly. What are your thoughts on diagnosis and management?

Q12

A 70-year-old widow who, at least until 2 years ago, was known by her general practitioner to be perfectly well, capable and self-reliant, has been noticed by her neighbours to be doing things such as leaving the door open, leaving the gas on and not taking care of her flat. You are asked by the general practitioner to see her on a home visit. How would you assess and manage this case?

Q13

A 55-year-old businessman had a myocardial infarction two weeks ago and is currently in the coronary care unit. The cardiologist has called a psychiatrist because the patient is very depressed and not eating. What advice would you give?

Q14

You are called as an independent psychiatrist on behalf of the Mental Health Act Commission, to give a second opinion on a treatment plan for a patient detained under Section 3 of the Mental Health Act 1983. The patient is refusing all treatment. He is a 35-year-old accountant who was admitted in a severely depressed state two months after the death of his boyfriend from severe pneumonia. He has marked psychomotor retardation and is refusing to eat. His consultant has suggested the following treatment plan: (1) electroconvulsive therapy followed by antidepressants; (2) HIV-antibody testing and appropriate treatment depending on the result. What would you do?

Q15

An 8-year-old boy is referred to you by his general practitioner. His parents are worried because the teacher said that he has not been talking at school for 2 months. How would you assess and manage this case?

Q16

A 21-year-old man with hydrocephalus who is wheelchair-bound is referred to you by his physician. He has been complaining of headaches and has frequent irritable outbursts. There is no identifiable physical problem that could be causing the headaches. The physician requests psychiatric assessment. What would you do?

Q17

A 45-year-old man, father of two children, is referred to you by his general practitioner, complaining that he has become impotent. His relationship with his wife has been deteriorating and he does not want her involved in his treatment. How would you manage this case?

Q18

A 28-year-old unemployed man, who admits he has been a heroin addict for years, comes to the accident and emergency department. He has been feeling depressed and physically unwell over the last few days. In the past, he attended a drug dependence clinic irregularly but gave up after a short while. He last saw a doctor some years ago, but now feels that he needs help. How are you going to help him?

Q19

An 11-year-old boy is brought to the accident and emergency department by his mother. She found him trying to cut his throat with a kitchen knife and managed to remove the knife from him, but not before he had made quite a deep cut. There have been some disciplinary problems at school. Over the last week, the child has been truanting from school, for the first time. They are a middle class family and are very disappointed and upset with him. There was a major family quarrel over the issue the night before his self-injurious behaviour.

The casualty officer requests a psychiatric assessment after suturing the wound. How would you deal with the situation?

Q20

A 50-year-old man is brought to the outpatient clinic by his daughter, who says she is fed up with his phone calls saying that the neighbours are plotting to kill him. He says he knows this is so because they have painted their door red in preparation. What action would you take?

Q21

A 19-year-old university student whose performance is falling is referred to you by his general practitioner. He complains of having persistent dreams of a burning football stand. What are your thoughts?

Q22

A 33-year-old school teacher, who has a 10-year history of recurrent episodes of mild depression is referred to you by her general practitioner, who feels she will benefit from psychotherapy. How will you assess her and what will your recommendation be?

Q23

A 15-year-old girl, whose grandmother died 3 months ago, is performing poorly at school. Recently, she started manifesting behavioural problems, both at school and at home. What are your thoughts about the possible reasons for this change in behaviour, and how would you deal with the problem?

Q24

You are called to see a 22-year-old stockbroker who is on remand and in custody for theft. The prison doctor reports that he has started behaving in a 'bizarre' manner, and is concerned about him. How do you go about assessing this man and what recommendations would you make?

Q25

As the liaison psychiatrist, you are asked to see a 24-year-old man who has been admitted to the general surgical ward for observation because of nausea, vomiting, constipation and acute abdominal pain. He has become very restless and violent. No previous psychiatric history has been elicited. A routine specimen of urine taken earlier in the day turned almost black on standing. How will you manage the violence and what other investigations would you carry out?

Q26

A 3-year-old boy with no physical abnormalities is referred to you by the paediatrician. Over the last year, his parents have noticed that he has had problems speaking and his behaviour is different from that of other children of his age. How would you assess this child?

Q27

A 24-year-old married woman with no previous psychiatric history is referred to you 2 weeks after the delivery of her first child. She was well for the first 10 days, after a normal delivery, and then began to complain that her pregnancy and delivery were broadcast on television, that journalists were pursuing her and that there were hidden devices in the house monitoring her behaviour. She also expressed feelings of guilt and appeared confused. How would you manage this patient?

Q28

A 40-year-old accountant who had a road traffic accident 2 years ago now complains of tiredness, irritability, low sex drive, dizziness and headaches. He sustained a minor blow on the head but did not lose consciousness during the road traffic accident. He has taken steps to sue the other driver. What is he suffering from? Will financial compensation alter his symptoms?

Q29

A 30-year-old teacher with no history of psychiatric disorder comes to see you at the outpatients' clinic. Her mother suffers from manic-depressive psychosis, and she wants to know her risks of having the illness. She is engaged to be married. Both she and her fiancé are worried about her passing the illness on to their children. How would you counsel them?

Q30

You are requested by the court to assess and advise on the future management of a 32-year-old single woman, from your catchment area, who has been charged with arson. She has a history of previous arson and is possibly subnormal. How would you assess her and advise on her management?

Q31

A 38-year-old shopkeeper was admitted to your ward 3 months ago for the treatment of a severe episode of depression. He has been treated with dothiepin 100 mg/day for the first seven weeks, and amitryptiline 200 mg/day for the rest of his admission, but has shown minimal improvement. He remains retarded, with delusions of guilt, and his business is suffering as a result of his illness.
A. What would you do? **B.** Do you think the patient has resistant depression? If so, how would you manage it?

Q32

A 22-year-old student is referred to you by the plastic surgeon. She thinks her nose is deformed, and says that this was the reason why her boyfriend left her. She now wants her nose operated on. There is, in fact, a minor defect, although the surgeon does not think her nose is grossly deformed. How will you advise her?

Q33

The general practitioner rings you up about a 65-year-old woman, living at home, who has become confused. The family do not want you to see her. How would you deal with it?

Q34

A 24-year-old nurse is referred to you. She started to wash her hands repeatedly about 6 weeks ago, following an unexpected and tragic death in the ward. How would you manage this case?

Q35

You are asked by a consultant in anaesthetics to see a colleague of his who is performing poorly at work. The theatre nurses have complained that in the mornings he is tremulous and there is always the smell of alcohol on his breath. At lunchtime, he insists on having 'a pint' in the pub. At social gatherings; he is always drunk and argumentative with his wife. How would you manage this problem?

Q36

You, as the liaison psychiatrist, are asked to see a 16-year-old girl in the casualty department. She took 80 tablets of paracetamol the previous evening, after a quarrel with her boyfriend. The house officer tells you that her paracetamol levels are low and that she is ready for discharge. She has made threats to kill herself, on previous occasions after minor quarrels or upsets. How will you advise the medical team?

Q37

You, as the liaison psychiatrist, are called by the general physician to see a 45-year-old married man recently admitted to his ward for the treatment of Hodgkin's disease. The patient is very difficult to control and is refusing to accept medication. Would you treat him against his will?

Q38

A 27-year-old single woman who works as a civil servant has been sending love letters to her superior, who in fact barely knows her and is feeling apprehensive about her attitude. The medical adviser informed her general practitioner, and she was finally referred to your outpatients' clinic. How would you assess this case?

Q39

A 37-year-old man with chronic schizophrenia, with no evidence of acute symptoms, has wandered in on a cold day to the accident and emergency department. He has frostbite and says he was discharged from a long-stay ward 2 months ago, having been there for 6 years. He has no friends or relatives. **A.** How will you arrange for his care? **B.** What is the likely cause for his frostbite?

Q40

You are asked to see the parents of a child with Down's syndrome who are planning to have another child. What advice will you give them?

Q41

A 30-year-old single librarian comes to your outpatient clinic asking for a sex change operation. He has a low sex-drive and says he has known from the age of 7 that he was of the wrong sex. How will you advise him and what would you do?

Q42

A 35-year-old homosexual man with a history of alcoholism and epilepsy, who has been in prison many times, is referred to you from prison with recent onset of fainting attacks. What is your differential diagnosis and management?

Q43

A 19-year-old girl from the country, who has never lived away from home, has recently taken a job as an au pair in the city, and is going to evening classes in dramatics. She has started to complain about her figure and feels she is obese and ugly. Her employers have noticed that she gets sick after every meal that they have together, and that on occasion large amounts of food have disappeared from the refrigerator. What are your thoughts on the diagnosis and possible aetiological factors? How would you manage her?

Q44

A 50-year-old housewife, complaining of abdominal pain for many years, is referred to you by her general practitioner. She was fully investigated and no physical abnormality was found. She comes for her appointment at the outpatients' clinic, but does not understand why she should see a psychiatrist. What would you do?

Q45

You are asked by the orthopaedic team to see a 57-year-old man, who had to undergo surgery under general anaesthesia three days ago for a fractured femur, after having fallen down a staircase. Over the last few hours, he has become very disturbed and violent and has had one epileptic fit. Earlier, he was complaining of poor memory, nausea and double vision. When you are assessing him, you demonstrate conjugate horizontal nystagmus and a sixth nerve palsy. What are the various diagnostic possibilities and how would you manage him?

Q46

A 43-year-old single teacher, with no previous psychiatric history, is referred to you by her general practitioner after investigation of her complaints of chest pain and headaches, in the course of which no pathology has been found. Her symptoms started about two years ago following the death of her mother, with whom she used to live. Previously a lively and sociable person, she lost interest in her friends and assumed a number of extra responsibilities at the school, with no time left for leisure or other activities. How would you counsel her?

Q47

You are referred a family who have recently moved into the area. The 15-year-old son with mental retardation, who lives with his parents, is showing increasing interest in sex. For the first time, he has exposed himself in a local shop. His parents are very concerned and upset. What would you do?

Q48

A general practitioner refers a 24-year-old shop assistant to you with a 5-year history of falling, with convulsions. She has been investigated for epilepsy without a firm conclusion, and the general practitioner suggests that there may be some doubts about the 'genuineness' of her presentation. How would you proceed?

Q49

A 31-year-old bus driver working in London is referred to you. Over the last few months, he stopped his bus a number of times while crossing Waterloo Bridge, thinking that he had a heart attack. On two occasions, he was taken to the accident and emergency department of the nearest hospital, but was found to be physically fit. He is now afraid of driving and is thinking of giving up his job. During the attacks, he has chest pain and feels breathless, and fears that he is going to die. How would you manage this case?

Q50

You are asked to assess an elderly woman in sheltered accommodation. She has had over 20 admissions over the last 35 years for being either depressed or elated, despite being on drugs continuously. The staff say that her behaviour is disturbed – she is dressing bizarrely, using excessive make-up and approaching the male residents inappropriately. How would you manage the situation?

Q51

You are seeing a 45-year-old woman with schizophrenia for a routine 2 monthly appointment in your outpatient clinic. She has been on depot neuroleptics for many years, and has recently started a part-time job after a break in employment for 15 years. You notice a twitch in the corner of her mouth but she not complained of it. What will you do?

Q52

You are called to see a 17-year-old girl, admitted to a surgical ward after a road traffic accident (RTA), during which she fractured her clavicle. In the last 12 hours, she has become acutely psychotic and will not allow people to touch her, saying they are going to rape her. While talking to her mother, you discover that she had been raped, exactly a year ago. What are your thoughts on diagnosis and management?

Q53

As the duty consultant, you are requested by the duty social worker to visit a local residential home over the weekend to see a 35-year-old resident with Down's syndrome who has recently moved in. He has become increasingly withdrawn and has not been talking to anyone for a day. He has also not been eating very well for a few weeks, and has lost weight. How will you deal with this request?

Q54

A 30-year-old woman who is now 11-weeks pregnant is referred to you by her general practitioner because she insists that she has vaginal herpes, although she was thoroughly examined and no pathology was found. She has always been a very religious and moral person and, five years ago, was admitted to a psychiatric hospital because 'God was talking to her'. At present, she is not being seen by a psychiatrist. How would you manage this case?

Q55

A 46-year-old married man is referred to you by his general practitioner. Over the last year or so, he has been feeling anxious, depressed and apathetic. He feels his thinking has become muddled, and is finding it difficult to keep his business under control. The general practitioner reports that the patient flicks his fingers intermittently and has abnormal facial movements. His father died in a psychiatric hospital. What are your thoughts about this case?

Q56

A 44-year-old social worker comes to you for advice. She has been on lithium for 5 years and wants to stop treatment. She had two attacks of hypomania and one of depression before she was started on lithium. What would you tell her?

Q57

Both you, and a general practitioner, have seen and felt it necessary to admit compulsorily a 69-year-old woman living in a nursing home. She has a long history of manic depressive illness and is very disturbed. She has left the nursing home and could not be traced when the social worker went to see her. Social workers, having made every effort to interview her, refuse to make an application for compulsory admission. How would you deal with the problem?

Q58

A 45-year-old barrister was admitted 4 days ago to the orthopaedic ward, having sustained multiple injuries in a car accident. He is now very disturbed and uncontrollable. You are called in as the duty liaison psychiatrist to see him. What would you do?

Q59

A 25-year-old male patient was discharged from your ward 2 weeks after a short admission. He was found to have no formal psychiatric disorder. He phones you and says he is going to commit suicide. What will you do?

Q60

A young male homosexual patient, admitted to a medical ward for an undiagnosed condition, is reported to be depressed. The registrar requests you to see him urgently, as he has been threatening to kill himself and has attempted to slash his wrists. He was smearing his blood and spitting all over the ward, and has refused to consider HIV testing. The staff have managed to quieten him down, but are unsure of what to do next. The other patients on the ward are threatening to discharge themselves unless he is moved. How would you manage the problem?

Answers

A1

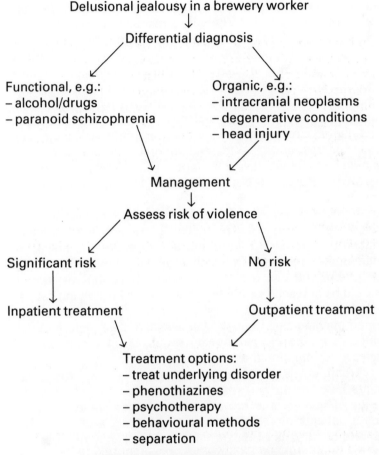

Delusional jealousy in a brewery worker
↓
Differential diagnosis

Functional, e.g.:
– alcohol/drugs
– paranoid schizophrenia

Organic, e.g.:
– intracranial neoplasms
– degenerative conditions
– head injury

Management
↓
Assess risk of violence

Significant risk

No risk

Inpatient treatment

Outpatient treatment

Treatment options:
– treat underlying disorder
– phenothiazines
– psychotherapy
– behavioural methods
– separation

SAFEGUARD AGAINST VIOLENCE

It is not unusual for patients with pathological jealousy to deny any problems when seen and to resist all interventions. The interview should, therefore, be handled very tactfully, and the first step is to secure the patient's confidence, or to start to do so. In the history, it is important to know how the belief of infidelity evolved and under what circumstances;

how firmly the belief is held; and whether the patient has other related beliefs (e.g. that his wife is plotting to infect him with venereal disease). One should determine what measures he takes to elicit evidence of his wife's infidelity, how resentful he feels and whether he has contemplated any acts of revenge against her or her imaginary or real lover. If the person he believes to be her lover is real, is that person aware of the situation? The wife's response to the patient's accusations and any investigative behaviour, as well as his response, to her behaviour in turn, should be carefully assessed. If there has been any history of violence, a careful account should be obtained of the circumstances under which it occurred and whether any injury was inflicted. If there is no history of actual violence it is important to find out under what circumstances she felt scared of the patient, and how she responded. A careful marital and sexual history should be obtained. It is important to see the patient's wife on her own, in order to obtain objective information about his condition.

Next, it is important to establish the fact that he has delusional jealousy, i.e. his belief in his wife's infidelity is indeed delusional in nature and that he holds the belief on inadequate grounds. Delusional or morbid jealousy is a *symptom*, and can occur in a variety of conditions. Mood should be assessed carefully, whatever the underlying cause, as patients are often miserable, irritable and angry, and their mood may indicate the risk of violence. A clear picture of the patient's premorbid personality should be obtained, as this helps in formulating the prognosis.

Treatment is often difficult, particularly since most patients lack insight and resent interference. There is a wide range of severity and risk of violence in this condition, with some patients needing outpatient care only, and others requiring conditions of maximum security. It may be possible to manage him as an outpatient. Inpatient management would be indicated if accurate assessment is not possible as an outpatient, if there is severe social and/or functional impairment, or if there is a significant risk of violence. Compulsory admission and treatment under the Mental Health Act may be necessary under these circumstances. If violence is one of the reasons for admission, adequate measures for security should be taken, including prevention of absconding by the patient. If the risk of him seriously harming his wife is significant if he absconds, a forensic opinion should be sought, with a view to managing him in a regional secure unit or a special hospital. Any underlying problem should be fully treated. Phenothiazine treatment may be effective, even in the absence of any underlying problems. Supportive psychotherapy may be helpful if there are underlying neurotic or personality problems. If there are sexual or marital problems, specific therapy for these problems should be offered, at the appropriate time. Behavioural techniques, such as teaching the patient's wife to respond in a manner that reduces aggression can be useful. A confession of infidelity only serves to accentuate the problem, and could precipitate serious violence. His wife should be advised against this. It is important that his wife is given adequate support and help throughout. An inadequate and sensitive premorbid personality, no clear underlying diagnosis and longstanding duration of the problem indicate a poor prognosis. Separation should be advised if there is a clear risk of violence and/or the response to treatment and prognosis is poor. The risk of violence should not be underestimated, as pathological jealousy is a significant factor in serious crime, especially homicide.

FURTHER READING

Mowat R R 1966 Morbid jealousy and murder. Tavistock, London

Mullen P E, Maack L 1985 Jealousy, pathological jealousy and aggression. In: Farrington D P, Gunn J (eds) Aggression and dangerousness. Wiley, London, pp 103–126

Shepherd M 1961 Morbid jealousy: some clinical and social aspects of a psychiatric symptom. Journal of Mental Science 107: 687–753

Tarrier N, Beckett R, Harwood S, Bishay N 1990 Morbid jealousy: a review and cognitive-behavioural formulation. British Journal of Psychiatry 157: 319–326

A2

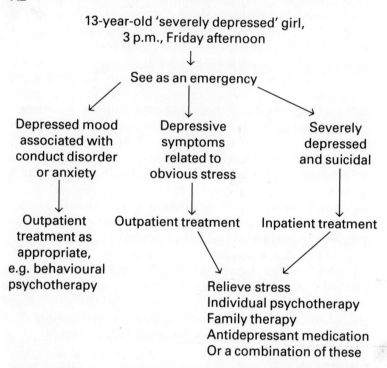

13-year-old 'severely depressed' girl,
3 p.m., Friday afternoon

↓

See as an emergency

Depressed mood
associated with
conduct disorder
or anxiety

Depressive
symptoms
related to
obvious stress

Severely
depressed
and suicidal

Outpatient
treatment as
appropriate,
e.g. behavioural
psychotherapy

Outpatient treatment

Inpatient treatment

Relieve stress
Individual psychotherapy
Family therapy
Antidepressant medication
Or a combination of these

Clearly, there is concern about this child. The first step is to find out why. Find out as much detail as possible from the social worker, e.g. how the girl came to her attention, and from other informants if possible. Arrange to see the girl as a matter of urgency, particularly as the weekend is approaching. The immediate decision would be whether the situation is sufficiently 'serious' as to warrant admission for further investigation and treatment. This decision will depend on information from the school, general practitioner, and parents/carers, as well as examination of the child.

A 13-year-old girl with severe depression is likely to have a history of previous episodes of depression, poor family care or institutional care, parental disruption and previous suicide attempts. There may also be evidence of behavioural disturbance, such as running away from home, truanting, hostility, rebelliousness and delinquency. All of these should be explored gently and carefully.

Depressed mood in children is commonly associated with other psychiatric symptoms and disorders, and a careful history and examination should establish whether this is a depressive disorder or not.

Depressive disorder is uncommon in children. Sadness and misery, often related to stress, are not uncommon and may be related to conduct disorders and neurotic conditions. Psychotic depression is commoner after puberty, and examination of her mental state may reveal longstanding sadness, feelings of guilt and self-blame, sleep disturbance, suicidal thoughts and/or psychomotor retardation.

Treatment depends on the foregoing assessment and the environment. If her condition is obviously related to stress, this should be removed or modified. The initial therapeutic aim should be to ensure her safety. If she is severely depressed and a serious suicide risk, she will have to be admitted and treated as an inpatient.

If the decision is made to admit, but the parents do not agree that the girl be admitted, the social worker could apply to the magistrate to make a place of safety order for up to 28 days. If there is no indication for admission, the patient can be managed as an outpatient. Treatment options include family therapy, individual psychotherapy, drug treatment or a combination of these. If drug treatment is judged necessary, antidepressants, such as imipramine, amitriptyline or dothiepin, may be used in adult doses. There is the possibility that there is no psychiatric problem, but the child needs to be removed from the home environment, e.g. for sexual abuse. In that case, the social worker may apply for a care order or a place of safety order. It is usual even in these circumstances for the patient and the family to be offered some form of counselling or family therapy.

FURTHER READING

Angold A 1988 Childhood and adolescent depression: 1 epidemiological and aetiological aspects. British Journal of Psychiatry 152: 601–617

Angold A 1988 Childhood and adolescent depression: II research in clinical populations. British Journal of Psychiatry 153: 476–492

Puig-Antich J, Gittelman R 1982 Depression in childhood and adolescence. In: Paykel E S (ed) Handbook of affective disorders. Churchill Livingstone, Edinburgh

A3

70-year-old woman with a history of depression and long-term use of benzodiazepines

A. Assessment:

- insomnia (detailed pattern, regularity/fluctuations)
- past history: depression/bereavement
- current physical problems
- social situation, daily routines.

B. Assessment for withdrawal from benzodiazepines.
   Risks: Benefits:

- severe withdrawal   - patient's satisfaction
- recurrence of depressive   - improvement of cognitive
  illness.   functions.
- rebound insomnia.

C. Benzodiazepine withdrawal management:

- switching to a long-acting benzodiazepine
- prescription of antidepressants
- gradual reduction of the dose of the benzodiazepine
- associated measures (e.g. behavioural treatment, anxiety management).

This is an elderly woman with a long history of benzo-diazepine use and sleep disturbance, who has been treated for depression in the past. Her history of depression and bereavement should be carefully explored, especially because she was started on lorazepam after her husband's death.

In your assessment, you would be looking particularly for factors which may complicate her withdrawal from lorazepam. These can include a physical illness, a psychiatric illness, or social problems, such as the absence of adequate support. Her complaints may be part of a recurrence of her depressive illness.

Even if she is not currently depressed, this lady has an increased risk of developing a severe withdrawal reaction on discontinuation of the benzodiazepine because of her long-term use of lorazepam, her age and her previous history of depressive illness. Withdrawal symptoms could include increased anxiety, agitation, rebound insomnia, somatic complaints of flu-like feelings, depersonalisation and derealisation, perceptual symptoms like visual hallucinations, strange taste in her mouth and feelings of motion. In this patient, there would be an increased risk of development of a severe psychotic depressive illness in view of her previous history of depression requiring electroconvulsive therapy. Psychomotor, cognitive and memory impairment are associated with long-term use of benzodiazepines and these functions may improve after discontinuation. The risks and benefits of withdrawal should be clearly explained. Social and environmental factors must be explored in order to ensure that the patient has maximum support during and after withdrawal.

Abrupt discontinuation must be avoided, especially because short-acting compounds such as lorazepam are associated with more severe withdrawal reactions. A sensible strategy would be to initiate a regime of sedating antidepressants and change the patient to a long-acting benzodiazepine (1 mg of lorazepam to 10 mg of diazepam). This would be followed by reducing the dose cautiously under regular supervision. Withdrawal may vary from weeks to several months, during which period she should be monitored for complications, especially a re-emerging depressive or even a psychotic illness.

Hospitalisation may be necessary if the risk of severe withdrawal symptoms, i.e. development of psychosis, is high or if there are complicating physical and social factors. If she is managed as an outpatient, the clinician should be available in order to allay her anxiety and to reassure her that some of the symptoms that she is experiencing are to be expected and will diminish with time. Behavioural treatment, such as anxiety management, may be of help.

In this patient, however, because of the significant risk of serious withdrawal-related problems, continuing her on this dose of lorazepam may be the most appropriate course of action. Provided that she never repeats or exceeds this dose, she should be reassured and advised to continue on the medication.

FURTHER READING

Dunbar G C, Perera M H, Jenner F A 1989 Patterns of benzodiazepine use in Great Britain as measured by a general population survey. British Journal of Psychiatry 155: 836–841

Higgitt A C, Lader M H, Fonagy P 1985 Clinical management of benzodiazepine dependence. British Medical Journal 291: 688–690

Kraupl Taylor F 1989 The damnation of benzodiazepines. British Journal of Psychiatry 154: 697–704

Lader M H 1988 Benzodiazepine dependence. International Review of Psychiatry 1: 149–165

Noyes R Jr, Garvey M J, Cook B L, Perry P J 1988 Benzodiazepine withdrawal: a review of the evidence. Journal of Clinical Psychiatry 49: 382–389

A4

There are two parts to this question: (A) dealing appropriately and professionally with requests for court reports; and (B) making a psychiatric assessment of a person who is to appear in court for indecent exposure.

A.   Request for a report:

– Must be a written request.
– The solicitor is obliged to supply details of the offence and any relevant information he may have.
– The psychiatrist writing the report must gather further relevant information from other sources, e.g. hospital and social service records, witness statements, probation services, etc., and study it thoroughly before seeing the client.
– More than one interview may be needed with the client, and the client must be willing to participate in the assessment. He is obliged to participate only if the court or prosecution requests a report.

The telephone request made in this case is, therefore, *not adequate* and the solicitor should be asked to forward a written request with relevant information.

B.   The second part of the question concerns assessment of the client and his offence. Indecent exposure first occurring at this age could be secondary to stress, depression, drug or alcohol use or organic brain disease (e.g. dementia). The client should be carefully assessed for the presence of any underlying physical, psychiatric or sexual problems. If there

have been previous offences, details of these
tained. The precipitant to each of the epis
assessed. Did the offence take place in a pub..
high risk of detection, or did the client take prec...
against being discovered? Have there been other forms of ab
normal sexual behaviour? His sexual response during the
offence should be assessed. Sexual excitement and mastur-
bation is usually associated with sexual aggression and lack
of guilt. The prognosis is poorer in these cases. Lack of a
sexual response and prominent feelings of guilt are associated with a better prognosis, and are usually seen in timid,
immature men. The effects of his offence on his personal life
and his work should be assessed. Will his wife/partner and
family be supportive during his treatment or have they re-
jected him as a result of the offence?

When writing the court report, the following essential
points need to be made:

- Whether the defendant has any form of mental disorder.
- Whether the defendant is fit to plead and stand trial.
- Whether he was capable of forming intent at the time of the
  offence.
- The treatment options open if there is an underlying treatable disorder. If the problem is exhibitionism, then a brief
  account of treatment options available, such as group or individual psychotherapy and various behaviour therapies
  (orgasmic reconditioning, aversion therapy, covert sen-
  sitisation, social skills training, etc.) should be mentioned,
  as well as where and when the treatment can be given.
- The prognosis. If there is an underlying medical or psychiatric condition, then the prognosis is that of this condition.
  80% of first-time sexual offenders do not re-offend in the
  first 5 years following their offence. The prognosis is poorer
  in those who repeatedly offend, and in those who derive
  sexual excitement from indecent exposure.

FURTHER READING

Bluglass R 1979 The psychiatric court report. Medicine, science and the law
19: 121–129

Brownell K D, Barlow D H 1980 The behavioural treatment of sexual
deviation. In: Goldstein A, Foa E B (eds) Handbook of behavioural
interventions. John Wiley, New York

ʋoth G 1973 Exhibitionism, sexual violence and paedophilia. British Journal of Psychiatry 122: 705–710

Snaith P, Bennett G 1990 Exhibitionism, indecent exposure, voyeurism and frottage. In: Bluglass R, Bowden P (eds) Principles and practice of forensic psychiatry. Churchill Livingstone, Edinburgh

A5

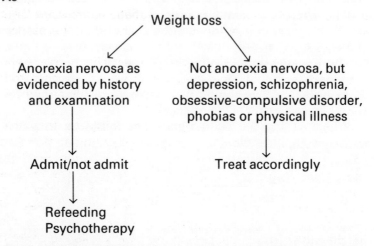

The immediate decision to be made is whether, on assessment, this is a case of anorexia nervosa or whether the anorexia is symptomatic of some other condition.

Of crucial importance in the history are previous episodes of excessive/very little eating, preoccupation with food, cooking, body size and weight, depression or amenorrhoea, as well as the patient's attitude to eating, weight, pregnancy, her family, etc. Similarly, features in the family history which would support a diagnosis of anorexia would be a family history of anorexia, high parental expectations, and family problems such as enmeshment, described by Minuchin. Physical examination may reveal signs of malnutrition, oedema, dehydration, bradycardia, hypotension, hypothermia or lanugo hair, or evidence of a physical cause for the weight loss.

Examination of her mental state should take into account the possible presence of depression, schizophrenia, obsessive-compulsive disorder and phobias – all of which can produce profound weight loss. Examination of her mental state may reveal a disorder of perception of body size and shape, i.e. a firm belief that she is fat or overweight despite the evidence.

If this is a case of anorexia nervosa, the treatment of choice is refeeding and psychotherapy. As this particular patient does not seem to have lost 40% of her body weight, it may be possible to treat her as an outpatient, provided there are no physical causes or family factors which necessitate admission.

Factors which could influence your decision to treat as an outpatient would be the patient's compliance, support from mother and her boyfriend, and a general practitioner who is known to the patient.

The first step in her management would be to gather more information from the general practitioner, previous notes, husband and any other informants. Further investigation should include haematology, biochemistry and tests of endocrine function. The refeeding programme is designed to ensure a weight increase of 1–2 kg/week with an intake of 3000 cal/day. A target weight is set as an average for the height and weight of the patient, preferably with the consent of the patient.

As the refeeding progresses, the patient will have to be carefully monitored to ensure that there is no vomiting or purging, and to ensure accurate recording of weight.

Supportive psychotherapy should be offered. Individual psychotherapy may be used with the target of improving self-identity and acknowledging sexuality. Family therapy may also be used, in conjunction with individual therapy. Cognitive therapy may also be offered as she is in the age range of patients who are said to respond better to this form of treatment.

FURTHER READING

Bhanji S, Mattingly D 1988 Medical aspects of anorexia nervosa. Wright, London

Minuchin S, Rosman B L, Baker L 1979 Psychosomatic families: anorexia nervosa in context. Harvard University Press, Cambridge

Mitchell J E 1986 Anorexia nervosa: medical and physiological aspects. In: Brownell K D, Foreyt J P (eds) Handbook of eating disorders: physiology, psychology and treatment of obesity, anorexia and bulimia. Basic Books, New York

Russell G F M 1981 The current treatment of anorexia nervosa. British Journal of Psychiatry 138: 164–166

Treasure J 1989 Eating disorders. Current Opinion in Psychiatry 2: 248–253

A6

A.

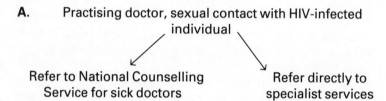

B.

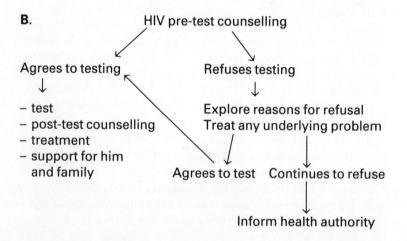

The issues raised in this question are:

– the duty of a doctor who feels there is a possibility that he is infected with HIV
– the duty of a doctor who believes a colleague is infected with the virus
– counselling for HIV testing and obtaining consent for the test.

– the issue of disclosure of test results to a third party without the consent of the patient.

The problem should be handled sensitively, and the doctor helped to make an informed decision. He should be allowed to talk about his concerns and express his feelings, before he is reminded about his moral and professional obligations. As he may find it easier to deal with doctors from outside his catchment area and his social circle, it may be best to refer him to the National Counselling Service for sick doctors. However, in a situation such as this the confidentiality that the service assures will not be maintained if the doctor refuses to have a test, or to disclose the results to the people concerned.

To begin with, he should see an experienced test counsellor and undergo HIV testing after pre-test counselling. Issues such as telling his wife are best tackled after he has decided whether or not to have the test, as he may well change his mind after pre-test counselling. It is important to identify reasons for his continuing refusal, such as an adjustment reaction or depression, and to deal with them first, before trying to persuade him to do what is expected of a responsible doctor in his situation. If he refuses to go ahead with either the counselling or the test after pre-test counselling, the following GMC guidelines should be brought to his notice:

1. Any doctor who thinks there is a possibility that he may have been infected with HIV *should* seek appropriate counselling and testing and, if found to be infected, should have regular medical supervision. He should seek specialist advice on the extent to which he should limit his professional practice in order to protect his patients and he *must* act on that advice. In this instance, it is the doctor's duty to seek counselling and testing and he stands the risk of losing his registration with the GMC, or having it curtailed, if he does not comply.

2. A doctor who has counselled a colleague, infected with HIV, to modify his or her professional practice in order to safeguard patients, and who is aware that this advice is not being followed, has a duty to inform an appropriate body that the colleague's fitness to practise may be seriously impaired.

There are guidelines about how a doctor can do this, and the issue is dealt with elsewhere. In this instance, if he cannot be persuaded to follow the GMC guidelines, one would have to inform the senior doctor appointed by the health authority to deal with issues of health in the doctors employed by the health authority. If the senior doctor is unable to persuade him to follow the guidelines, he should inform the general manager (GM). It then becomes the responsibility of the GM to take administrative action by invoking the health procedures of the health authority.

3. A third party cannot be informed of the results without the consent of the patient. There are grounds for such a disclosure only when there is a serious and identifiable risk to a specific individual, or a health care professional who, if not so informed, would be exposed to infection. In this case, it is likely that he will agree to disclose the results to his wife after the implications of his condition are discussed with him. He should be advised to take precautionary measures, even if he is HIV-negative, as the sample may have been taken before seroconversion. If he refuses to inform his wife after he is found to be HIV-positive and is continuing to have sexual intercourse with her, then it is the duty of the professionals involved in his care to ensure that she is informed. Depending on the situation, it may be you, the general practitioner or another health care professional who should tell her. In all other respects, it is his right to expect total confidentiality.

FURTHER READING

Advisory Committee on Dangerous Pathogens 1990 HIV – the causative agent of AIDS and related conditions. Second revision of guidelines. HMSO, London

General Medical Council 1988 HIV infection and AIDS: the ethical considerations. General Medical Council, London

Goldmeier D, Granville-Grossman K 1988 The clinical psychiatry of human immunodeficiency virus (HIV) infection. In: Granville-Grossman K (ed) Recent advances in clinical psychiatry, Vol 6, pp. 1–67

See also Q11, Q14, Q35 and Q60.

A7

Assessment of primary nocturnal enuresis: predisposing/pre-cipitating factors, e.g.:

- family history
- developmental delay
- large family with social problems
- events during period of establishing bladder control.

Treatment:

- fluid restriction
- toilet before bed/waking for toilet
- reducing criticism/rewarding success/star charts
- bell and pad
- drugs/other techniques.

Enuresis seems to be a familial developmental delay and the boy may be found to have a first-degree relative who has been enuretic. Other predisposing and precipitating factors should be looked for in his developmental history. Details of his birth (e.g. low birth weight), milestones (delays), behaviour and skills (e.g. features suggestive of a low IQ) will have to be obtained. Significant events during the period of establishing bladder control (e.g. birth of a sibling, moving to another place, separation from parents) may have occurred. The situation of the boy's family should be assessed. He may have a large family facing social and financial difficulties.

The boy's enuresis may be associated with a physical problem, and he should be investigated for conditions such as an urinary tract infection, diabetes, epilepsy or congenital anomalies.

Treatment of his enuresis would include the following:

A. If a physical illness is detected, treatment or referral for specialised management should be arranged. If no organic cause is found, measures such as restriction of fluid intake in the evenings, emptying the bladder before going to bed or waking him at night to take him to the toilet may be sufficient. The family should be encouraged to reduce critical attitudes and reward success. Simple behavioural techniques, such as star charts, can be used. If enuresis persists, the bell and pad method can be used. In this technique, the child sleeps on a pad which is electrically connected to a bell. When the pad becomes wet, the circuit is completed and the bell rings. This inhibits urination. The parents should wake him to empty his bladder in the toilet, remake his bed and reset the system.

B. The bell and pad technique is effective in two thirds of cases. One third of cases relapse after a year. However, response may take up to 2 months, and it often fails because the parents do not persist long enough, which is likely to be the case in this boy. The treatment may need to be continued for months. Failure to respond may be due to a physical or psychiatric disorder, or a recent stressful life experience. Family therapy and/or individual psychotherapy may be indicated.

New operant techniques, such as the dry bed method and the tangible reward with fading method, may be of help. Both methods include the bell and pad technique coupled with training programmes, and involve the whole family in a re-training exercise. In case enuresis persists, prescription of tricyclics (imipramine 25–50 mg at night) can give good results. However, the risks involved in using these drugs in young children must not be overlooked.

FURTHER READING

Kaplan S L, Breit M, Gauthier B et al 1989 A comparison of three nocturnal enuresis treatment methods. Journal of the American Academy of Child and Adolescent Psychiatry 28: 282–286

Shaffer D 1987 The development of bladder control. In Rutter M (ed) Developmental psychiatry. American Psychiatric Press, Washington, D.C., pp 129–137

A8

A. The cause of auditory hallucinations, particularly in a man of this age, may be either functional or organic.

The hallucinations may be part of late-onset schizophrenia, in which case it would be associated with other evidence of schizophrenia, or paraphrenia. Manic-depressive illness may be the reason for the hallucinations. Auditory hallucinations, though not as common as visual hallucinations, do occur in acute organic syndromes. Here, there is clouding of consciousness with changes in behaviour, slow muddled thinking, lability of mood and visual misperceptions.

The possible causes of acute organic syndrome in this patient would include:

- withdrawal of alcohol or anxiolytic-sedative drugs
- metabolic causes, such as uraemia, liver failure, cardiac failure, respiratory failure and electrolyte imbalance
- endocrine causes, such as hypoglycaemia
- intracranial tumours or other space-occupying lesions
- head injury
- cerebral infections such as encephalitis
- systemic infections such as pneumonia
- starvation or vitamin deficiency, e.g. thiamine
- drugs, such as digitalis, levodopa, bromocriptine, amantadine hydrochloride, sympathomimetic agents like decongestants, cimetidine, propranolol hydrochloride, anticholinergics like atropine and benztropine, amitryptiline hydrochloride and thioridazine, and disulfiram.

Deafness may be a cause or a contributing factor to this patient's auditory hallucinations and his odd behaviour.

B. The patient may have paraphrenia, although this is relatively uncommon and is more likely to occur in women than in men. It does occur more frequently in those living alone, and may be associated with deafness.

The first decision will have to be whether this man needs to be admitted to hospital or not. This will depend, firstly on whether he is able to continue living in the community or whether he is in any way at risk. Compulsory admission may be required if he refuses admission and his health or safety are at risk. Secondly, the decision to admit him may be dictated by the need to carry out further, more detailed, enquiries. These may be carried out as a day assessment or as a series of home assessments. The latter may be preferable if he has social support. Medication is usually necessary, and phenothiazines such as promazine or trifluoperazine may be used, but in reduced doses. The patient should also be referred to the local ENT specialist for assessment and the provision of a hearing aid.

A9

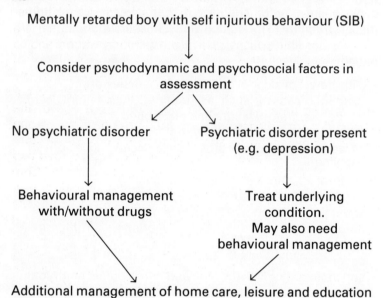

Mentally retarded boy with self injurious behaviour (SIB)

↓

Consider psychodynamic and psychosocial factors in assessment

No psychiatric disorder   Psychiatric disorder present (e.g. depression)

Behavioural management with/without drugs   Treat underlying condition. May also need behavioural management

Additional management of home care, leisure and education

The problem here is SIB of recent onset in a 6-year-old mentally retarded boy, preceded by his parents' divorce and a change in his mother's job commitments. The answer should cover assessment of SIB, assessment for psychiatric disorder and relevant psychosocial and psychodynamic factors. Similarly, the treatment plan must cover all aspects of his care at home, keeping in mind his mother's recent move to a full-time job.

Mention should be made of the need for a psychiatric history, including an accurate account of the onset and progression of his SIB, and details of any physical complications. Features that would alert one to the presence of depression or a psychotic illness in a mentally retarded person include a decline in level of functioning, social withdrawal, loss of interest in usual activities, a sad appearance and loss of appetite and sleep, emergence of unfamiliar, bizarre or inexplicable behaviour and psychomotor retardation. The effect of the SIB on the family should be carefully examined, as SIB can be used by the child to gain attention or to reduce tension in high-demand situations. Whatever the nature of the injuries, physical abuse by others in the family should be considered. It is essential that the mother and, if possible, the father are seen, to get a clearer picture of the family situation and to look for evidence of psychiatric and/or physical illness in them. The divorce may have been preceded by a particularly difficult period, and one should assess the tensions and problems at that time. The patient may have been one of the causes of marital disharmony, or could have been the reason for the couple trying to stay together in an unsatisfactory marriage, until the divorce. The family should be visited and seen together at home. Information should be obtained from other professionals involved – teachers, social worker, psychologist, family doctor and paediatrician – all of whom will need to be involved in the management. A careful physical examination and relevant investigations should be carried out, by a paediatrician if necessary. Complications, such as fractures, a subdural haematoma and infected wounds, should be looked for. Careful mental state examinations should be carried out, exploring specifically for signs of a psychosis, depression and/or intellectual deterioration. A detailed functional analysis of the boy's behaviour should be carried out, in order to work out a suitable behaviour modification programme.

The treatment would depend on the nature of the primary problem. Keeping in mind the recent onset of the behaviour, following significant changes in the family structure, it could be the manifestation of an adjustment reaction in the boy. Treatment would, in this case, concentrate on helping him and the family come to terms with the inevitable changes in their lifestyle, and offering appropriate practical and psychological support.

The treatment of SIB in this case would be mainly by behavioural modification. This should initially be tried at home, and hospital admission considered only if proper assessment is not possible as an outpatient, if any factors preclude home treatment, or if the SIB persists despite treatment. Positive and negative reinforcement can be used in the behaviour modification programme, for example increased attention or exemption from carrying out a task he does not like when he does not injure himself. If this does not work, positive reinforcement can be temporarily withdrawn and strategies such as placing the boy in a featureless room when he does injure himself can be used. This should be supplemented by protective measures. For example, if needed, a 'bubble helmet' can be used contingently for head banging. Other aversive techniques, such as withdrawal of privileges, can also be used. It is important that the entire family is familiar with the therapy and that it is used consistently. Fluphenazine, a D1 receptor blocker, seems to reduce SIB in Lesch-Nyhan syndrome, and may be useful in other forms of SIB. Lithium is often used, although there is little evidence to support its efficacy. More recently, opiate antagonists have been used, as endogenous opiods may have a role in the pathogenesis of SIB.

Other possible components of management include day care, family therapy, and support for the family in the form of relief admission and 'child minding' on some evenings. If the behaviour is manifest at school, the teacher should be involved in the programme.

The candidate should be familiar with the general principles of community care for the mentally handicapped, and be able to work out the most suitable strategy for the patient. However, the patient has been referred at the age of 6, and most of these measures may have been implemented by then.

FURTHER READING

Corbett J A 1985 Mental retardation: psychiatric aspects. In: Rutter M L, Hersov L (eds) Child psychiatry: modern approaches. Blackwell, Oxford, pp 661–668

Oliver C 1988 Self-injurious behaviour in people with a mental handicap. Current Opinion in Psychiatry 1: 567–571

A10

The most important task is to contact the patient.

The first step would be to check whether anybody has tried phoning him, if he is on the telephone. Has he been seen by friends or relatives in the last few days, or do they know his whereabouts? Attempts should be made to contact his general practitioner and social worker if he has one. Whether or not he has been seen by other people, it would still be important to do a home visit, preferably with his key worker or somebody else from the team who knows him well. The visit would serve to establish whether he is at home, the reason for his non-attendance, and any deterioration in his physical or mental state. He may have not attended because he has a physical illness, such as influenza, or he may have become profoundly depressed and withdrawn.

If he is at home, both physical and mental state examination should be carried out, as well as re-assessment of his living conditions. In particular, attention should be paid to his provision for food, heating arrangements and financial situation. If he does not appear to be at home, or does not answer the door, the neighbours may give some indication of when he was last seen. Several visits during the day may have to be made in order to find him in. If nobody has seen him in the last 3 days, and there is no reason to think that he has suddenly gone away to visit family or on holiday, the next step would be to request social services to gain entry to his home, using Section 135 of the Mental Health Act.

Under this section of the Act any approved social worker who has reasonable cause to believe that a person suffering from a mental disorder and (a) 'has been, or is being, ill-treated, neglected or kept otherwise than under proper control, or (b) is living alone and is unable to care for him/her self', can apply to a Justice of the Peace for a warrant. This warrant authorises a police officer, accompanied by a registered doctor and an approved social worker, to enter the person's premises, if necessary by force. The warrant also authorises the removal of the person, if appropriate, to a place of safety for a period of up to 72 hours.

Should the patient not be at home, and there is no indication of his whereabouts, he should be reported to the police as a missing person, whilst other enquiries are continued.

A 11

Young, frail man, agitated, aggressive, with needle marks, who responded readily to chlorpromazine

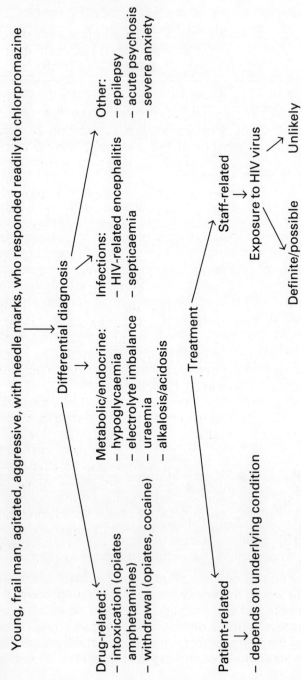

Differential diagnosis

Drug-related:
– intoxication (opiates amphetamines)
– withdrawal (opiates, cocaine)

Metabolic/endocrine:
– hypoglycaemia
– electrolyte imbalance
– uraemia
– alkalosis/acidosis

Infections:
– HIV-related encephalitis
– septicaemia

Other:
– epilepsy
– acute psychosis
– severe anxiety

Treatment

Patient-related
– depends on underlying condition

Staff-related

Exposure to HIV virus

Definite/possible
First aid measures
Regular testing
Counselling

Unlikely
Reassurance

A11

The presence of needle marks could suggest intravenous drug use, repeated injections for conditions such as diabetes, frequent blood transfusions, or dialysis. Any of the above could lead to complications that present as an acutely disturbed state. The poor physical condition of the man and his quick response to chlorpromazine should alert one to the possibility of opiate intoxication and debilitating physical conditions. On the other hand, the presence of needle marks should not prevent one from considering a functional psychosis.

Treatment here is both patient-directed and staff-directed. The first step is to obtain all relevant information for a complete assessment: from nursing and medical staff involved, the friends who brought him in, his general practitioner and past records if possible. If after waking up in the morning the patient remains disturbed, and an underlying psychiatric problem is present, he should be transferred to a psychiatric ward for further care. Admission may need to be under Section 2 of the Mental Health Act, if he refuses any assessment or treatment. The exact treatment will depend on the underlying cause and will not be discussed here. The candidate is advised to work out treatment for each of the diagnostic possibilities outlined in the flow diagram.

The staff members' concern here is quite clearly about the possibility of HIV infection. Though there is no evidence that infection can be transmitted by saliva, it is advisable that the staff member concerned report to his supervisor and to the occupational health department, who should be able to advise him on how to proceed. At the time of the injury, the wound should have been washed thoroughly with soap and water and bleeding encouraged in order to express any material deposited in the wound. The risk of exposure can be assessed if the HIV status of the patient can be obtained, both at the time of the injury and at regular intervals. However, this can only be done if he has agreed to pre-test counselling and if the result would materially improve his management. If it cannot be obtained and the patient is felt to be at increased risk of infection, or if the patient is HIV-positive, then it is advisable that the staff member is treated as potentially infected i.e. has professional counselling and is tested at regular intervals.

FURTHER READING

Advisory Committee on Dangerous Pathogens 1990 HIV – the causative
    agent of AIDS and related conditions. Second Revision of Guidelines.
    HMSO, London

Departments of Health 1990 Guidance for clinical health care workers:
    protection against infection with HIV and hepatitis viruses. HMSO,
    London

Jeffries D 1987 ABC of AIDS: control of infection policies. British Medical
    Journal 295: 33–35

See also Q6, Q14 and Q60

A12

This is an elderly woman who lives on her own and seems to
be suffering from cognitive impairment. Before making the
visit, it is important to obtain as much information as possible
from the general practitioner, family, etc. about her situation.
It would also be useful to know who the carers are, if there are
any. The general practitioner should be invited to accompany
you on the visit, and arrangements should be made to ensure
that the patient is kept at home and that somebody is available to give access to the flat. Although dementia seems to be
the most likely diagnosis on the limited information available,
a functional illness should also be considered. Information on
the course and severity of the woman's deterioration should
be gathered from her neighbours and relatives. The time and
mode of onset must be established, and her general practitioner may be able to provide details of her medical history
and physical state. Her activities and the way she has been
coping with her needs – mobility, physical disabilities, cooking and feeding, shopping, bills, financial affairs – and the
support on which she can count (e.g. family, neighbours,
social services) will have to be explored. However, it may be
difficult to obtain all the necessary information on a single
home visit.

The condition of her flat will indicate the extent of her
difficulties: for example, rotten food, rubbish on the floor, a
smell of urine and/or faeces and very poor hygiene may indicate severe deterioration. Individual cognitive impairments,

such as dyspraxia, agnosia and dysphasia, can be tested by tasks such as using the telephone or the oven, describing objects in the flat and naming people in photographs, i.e. activities of daily living, in contrast to hospital assessment which often uses artificial tests, such as copying drawings. The patient may be found be suffering from delirium (acute organic brain syndrome) related to a physical illness, and be in need of medical care; in this case she may have to be seen by a geriatrician first. Careful examination of her mental state may reveal depressive symptoms. If this is a depressive illness, the severity of the symptoms would suggest that it is a psychotic depression. It must be remembered that patients with dementia, especially early dementia, often exhibit depressive symptoms.

The next step is to determine whether or not this patient needs admission for further assessment and management. If this is necessary and she does not wish to be admitted, it must be established that she is sufficiently at risk (e.g. in terms of health, safety) to be admitted against her will.

Along with the medical and psychiatric measures which prove necessary, the patient must be assessed in detail for her level of functioning and self-care, and for her needs, both at present and in the future. Aspects such as the severity of her impairment, the suitability of her accommodation, the amount of care and supervision that she requires, the help that is available and the social or financial support she may need must be established by the multidisciplinary team.

The conclusion may be such that the patient can stay in the community provided that her safety and wellbeing are ensured. Local community services should be mobilised in a scheme which includes the general practitioner, a district nurse, social services, meals-on-wheels, home-help, laundry service, visits by a community psychiatric nurse, referral to a day-centre and follow-up as an outpatient. The appropriate 'package' depends on her needs. The patient could be referred to the local case management service, if available. If possible, her family should be encouraged to become involved in her care. Voluntary agencies such as the Alzheimer's Disease Society and Age Concern can prove invaluable.

If the patient cannot be safely cared for in the community, a nursing home or local authority residential care should be considered. If it is essential that she moves but she refuses to do so, a guardianship order may have to be organised by the social worker. Other arrangements (court of protection, power of attorney) may be necessary to protect the patient from financial risk.

The finding of profound deterioration, with behavioural disturbance, poor self-care and the absence of any support may require the patient's immediate admission to a psycho-geriatric ward as an inpatient, especially if it is clear that she would be at risk if left on her own. In these circumstances, she may have to be admitted under Section 2 of the Mental Health Act 1983.

FURTHER READING

Jacques A 1988 Understanding dementia. Churchill Livingstone, Edinburgh

Renshaw J 1987 Care in the community: individual care planning and case management. British Journal of Social Work 18: 79–105

A13

A 55-year-old man with a post-myocardial depression

Immediate management:
- physical treatment (ECT and/or anti-depressants)
- transfer to open ward
- mobilisation
- emotional support

Long-term management:
- supportive psychotherapy
- rehabilitation
- counselling/support for the family
- management type-A behaviour
- group psychotherapy

Information from the medical and nursing staff must be obtained about: the circumstances of admission of the patient (elective or emergency); the severity of the myocardial infarction (MI) and the treatment required (cardiac catheterisation and/or bypass surgery, medication); possible complications that may have occurred (arrhythmias, thromboembolism); and his physical state at present (mobilisation, short- and long-term prognosis). In his psychiatric history, it is important to know if he has been treated for an affective illness or has had depressive symptoms in the past.

A physical and neurological examination should be done, along with the careful assessment of his cognitive functions and mental state. Affective symptoms could develop due to metabolic dysfunction, drugs or cerebrovascular problems.

If the patient is severely depressed and found to be suicidal, or jeopardizing his life by refusing to eat or take his medication, electroconvulsive therapy (ECT) would be indicated. Antidepressants may be used concurrently with ECT and, if so, should be maintained for 6 to 9 months. However, cardiotoxicity, side-effects (e.g. anticholinergic) and interaction with other drugs (e.g. anti-hypertensive compounds) may be contraindications to their use. Second generation antidepressants, such as lofepramine (140–210 mg daily) or doxepin (75–300 mg daily), may be appropriate and administered in divided doses, since once-nightly dosage regimens are best avoided in this situation.

In MI, an increase in life stress often precedes illness, and predisposing/precipitating factors should be explored with the patient's family: financial threat or other pressure at work, difficulties at home, previous episodes of depression, or a behaviour pattern characterised by extremes of competitiveness, chronic sense of urgency and hostility (type A behaviour) may be found.

Symptoms of depression and anxiety following an MI may be related to social, financial or psychological problems and, in this context, the illness may have a particularly threatening or stressful meaning. The patient may well have denied early cardiac symptoms and delayed seeking treatment, all these having contributed to precipitate a state of helplessness and distress.

Should the patient's condition allow, he should be transferred from the coronary care unit (CCU) to an open ward, as intensive care units are high stress environments. His transfer from the CCU may lead to anxiety or depression, since he is likely to receive less attention/supervision and may feel more alone in the open ward. Therefore, the psychiatrist should work closely with the cardiology team, especially with medical nurses, in order to ensure adequate support. The importance of constant emotional support and reassurance from the earliest stage cannot be underestimated: short- and long-term predictors of recurrence of the MI and death include the level of anxiety/depression during and after hospitalisation, and the number of days spent in the coronary care unit. Early mobilisation and exercise training should be encouraged.

It is essential to ascertain the degree of psychological and social support that both the patient and his family need. Supportive psychotherapy as an outpatient, methods to reduce stress and manage type A behaviour (e.g. relaxation techniques) and a rehabilitation programme (e.g. changes in lifestyle, appropriate routine) should be implemented. Counselling and support for the patient's family is important. Group therapy may be helpful. If a group for spouses is available, his wife could participate. Family or marital therapy may be beneficial.

FURTHER READING

Appels A 1990 Mental precursors of myocardial infarction. British Journal of Psychiatry 156: 465–471

Frasure-Smith N, Prince R 1989 Long-term follow-up of the ischemic heart disease life stress monitoring program. Psychosomatic Medicine 51: 485–513

Mayou R, Hawton K 1986 Psychiatric disorder in a general hospital. British Journal of Psychiatry 149: 172–190

Raft D, Cohen-Cole S, Bird J 1982 Liaison psychiatry. In Cavenar J O, Brodie H K H (eds) Critical problems in psychiatry. J B Lippincott, Philadelphia, pp 422–453

A14

Second opinion on treatment plan for severely depressed
male refusing treatment, possibly HIV-infected.

Assess

– current physical and mental state and ability and willingness to give informed consent

Consult team

Evaluate treatment plan

Agree with ECT/anti-	Disagree with HIV testing.
depressant treatment	Advise pre-test counselling
– specify number of ECT	after improvement in
applications, dose range	mental state
of antidepressant and	
sign form	

The patient should be seen first for a complete psychiatric
assessment and the treatment plan evaluated independently.
The responsible medical officer or his deputy, a nurse and
one other professionally involved person must be consulted.
It is essential to determine whether or not the patient is capable of understanding the nature, purpose and likely effect of
the treatment and can give informed consent, *and* that the
treatment will alleviate or prevent a deterioration in the patient's condition. After the assessment, one may agree or
disagree with the treatment plan. Given the severity of the
depression, the patient's refusal to eat and the presence of
marked psychomotor retardation, it is clear that the patient
needs treatment which will lead to an improvement fairly
quickly. The team's decision to give him ECT and antidepressants is correct and one would agree with this. The number of
applications of ECT and the dose range of the antidepressants
should be specified.

HIV testing in this case is *not treatment*. Though knowing the HIV status of the patient will obviously help in the long-term management, it does not affect the immediate management. Moreover, the boyfriend may not have had AIDS-related pneumonia. If there is concern about the infectivity of the patient, precautionary measures could be taken even without a positive test result and, in this case, are probably advisable as the patient will be under general anaesthesia while undergoing ECT. The consultant was wrong to include HIV testing as part of the treatment plan here, and the team cannot justify proceeding with the testing, at present. It could be suggested that the patient is approached and counselled about the possibility of having the test after his mental state has improved and he is able fully to understand the implications of having the test, whatever the result. He should be counselled about the test by a trained counsellor, and the test carried out only if he gives his written consent.

FURTHER READING

Advisory Committee on Dangerous Pathogens 1990 HIV – the causative agent of AIDS and related conditions. Second revision of guidelines. HMSO, London

General Medical Council 1988 HIV infection and AIDS: the ethical considerations. General Medical Council, London

See also Q6 and Q60.

A15

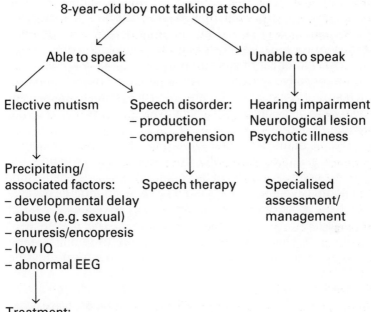

8-year-old boy not talking at school

Able to speak · Unable to speak

Elective mutism · Speech disorder: – production – comprehension · Hearing impairment / Neurological lesion / Psychotic illness

Precipitating/
associated factors:
– developmental delay
– abuse (e.g. sexual)
– enuresis/encopresis
– low IQ
– abnormal EEG

Speech therapy

Specialised
assessment/
management

Treatment:
– psychotherapy
– behaviour modification
– treatment of associated conditions

The first step of the assessment is to ascertain whether the child has previously spoken and, if so, his parents should be asked whether his speech was normal in form and content. If not, the nature of the abnormality must be ascertained. They may be able to clarify, for example, whether the child had difficulties with the production (e.g. articulation) or with the comprehension of language. If he had a history of not being able to speak, this could be associated with a severe mental handicap or a pervasive developmental disorder. Inability to speak may also be associated with neurological lesions, hearing impairment or a psychotic illness with thought disorder.

The child may talk normally in some situations (e.g. at home) and be mute in others (e.g. at school). If this is the case, and his ability to comprehend spoken language is unimpaired, then a diagnosis of elective mutism should be made.

Precipitating factors should be investigated. The boy may have stopped talking after starting or changing school. A stressful life experience may have occurred. A history of abuse, particularly sexual abuse, may be present. His milestones must be carefully assessed. Developmental delays (e.g. delayed onset of speech) may be found, along with features suggestive of a low IQ. An underlying speech handicap, such as stuttering, could be present. He may have enuresis or encopresis. In many cases, elective mutism is associated with an abnormal EEG.

Details of his behaviour should be obtained. He may be a shy and sensitive child who cries easily and is withdrawn from his peers. A history of temper tantrums, sulky behaviour and aggressiveness with strangers may be found. His parents may have a history of personality (aggressiveness, shyness) or psychiatric (e.g. depression) disorder. The presence of marital problems between the parents and the family dynamics (e.g. an overprotective mother, family distress) must be explored.

Management will depend on the findings of the assessment. For example, if a neurological or hearing problem is detected, referral for specialised assessment (e.g. audiological evaluation) and treatment should be arranged. If a speech disorder is detected, physical problems must be considered (e.g. malocclusion, defects in the tongue, respiratory dysfunction). Language function testing and referral for speech therapy may be indicated. Other conditions, such as enuresis, should be treated. Treatment of elective mutism can include individual psychotherapy, behaviour modification (e.g. using tangible rewards for talking) and social relearning. Family therapy may be indicated. The safety of the child must be ensured if evidence of sexual abuse is found, in which case the involvement of social services is essential. Elective mutism may take months to improve.

FURTHER READING

Frame C L, Matson J L 1987 Handbook of assessment in childhood psychopathology. Plenum Press, London

Wilkins R 1985 A comparison of elective mutism and emotional disorders in children. British Journal of Psychiatry 146: 198–203

A16

Headaches and irritable outbursts in a 21-year-old man with hydrochephalus could be due to

Functional problems, e.g.	Organic problems, e.g.	Behavioural problems, e.g.
– anxiety	– drugs	– related to frustration
– depression	– cognitive	– related to life events
– hypomania	impairment	

OR a combination of the above

It has already been made clear that there is no identifiable physical cause for this patient's headaches, otherwise the first step would have been to establish whether his shunt is blocked.

The first step in the assessment is to get a detailed account of the presenting problems. How long he has had the headaches and been irritable; whether they are related in any way; how long they last for; whether there are any apparent precipitants; whether there are any other related symptoms, etc. He may have had similar episodes in the past. Have there been any changes in his life circumstances of late, such as change of accommodation or care-givers or events in the family? Have there been any other major life events?

A history of the patient's physical development and disabilities is important. He may have spina bifida, which is not infrequently associated with hydrocephalus, and urinary incontinence. He may have had frequent surgical intervention for maintenance of CSF drainage (shunts), and he may also have had frequent hospitalisations for other reasons, such as infections, with repeated disruptions to his life. He may be continuing to receive medication, and it is important to know what this is. His educational history should be explored with details of the type of school he went to, i.e. special school or ordinary school, how much school he missed because of ill health, and level of educational attainment. Has the patient been able to continue his education, or work in open employment, or sheltered employment, and if so how has he coped there? In terms of his psychosocial history, it is important to know whether there have been any problems, because these may be the underlying cause of his irritability. He may have a previous history of psychiatric disturbance or of epilepsy. It would be important to know about his social and financial circumstances and whether there are any problems in these areas.

The patient's knowledge of his disabilities and the extent to which he has come to terms with these are important to establish.

Examination of his mental state may reveal signs of anxiety, depression or hypomania, abnormal beliefs or experiences and/or cognitive impairment. Further investigation would include getting information from other informants, e.g. mother and the general practitioner, as well as assessment of his home circumstances. More detailed cognitive testing may be required, and this should be compared with his previous cognitive assessments.

Treatment will depend on the cause. If it is a purely behavioural problem related to inability to tolerate frustration, then the most appropriate treatment would be behavioural management. This could be combined with counselling, particularly over sexual difficulties. This could be arranged with the Committee on Sexual and Personal Relationships of the Disabled (SPOD), the organisation which offers help with sexual matters to the disabled. Major psychiatric disorder such as hypomania or depression should be treated with neuroleptics or antidepressants. Drugs should be used with caution because of the increased risk of side-effects in people with mental impairment, e.g. development of extrapyramidal symptoms at relatively small doses with neuroleptics, and severe anticholinergic effects with antidepressants. He may also need help with changing his accommodation, structuring his daytime activities, organising his finances and developing a social network.

FURTHER READING

Ghaziuddin M 1988 Behavioural disorder in the mentally handicapped: the role of life events. British Journal of Psychiatry 152: 683–686

Russell J A O 1989 Community living. Current Opinion in Psychiatry 2: 618–622

A17

A 45-year-old man with secondary impotence in the setting of marital disharmony

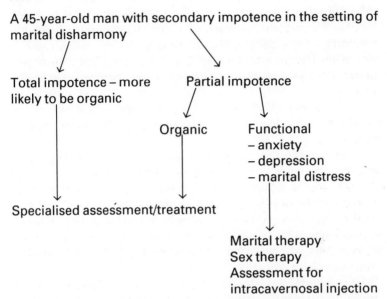

Total impotence – more likely to be organic

Partial impotence

Organic

Functional
– anxiety
– depression
– marital distress

Specialised assessment/treatment

Marital therapy
Sex therapy
Assessment for
intracavernosal injection

The first step is to determine the nature of the patient's impotence (erectile or ejaculatory). If he has erectile impotence, it must be ascertained whether he is unable to achieve an erection in any situation (total impotence), or if he is able to achieve full erection in some situations but not in others (partial impotence).

The history of total impotence is more likely to be associated with an organic cause. An example of this would be diabetes or alcohol abuse. Anticholinergic or anti-hypertensive drugs may also cause impotence. Other causes of impotence include: cardiovascular problems, renal problems, neurological disorders, hypothalamic/pituitary dysfunction and trauma.

Even if the patient has partial impotence, an organic cause should not be discounted. It is important to establish whether he has another partner with whom he is not impotent. He should be examined for a concurrent psychiatric illness (e.g. depression, anxiety). In this patient, his symptoms seem to be related to marital distress. The situation at home should be explored, and the patient encouraged to talk about his marital difficulties.

Specialised assessment and treatment would be required if an underlying organic condition is detected. If he is found to have partial impotence associated with a psychiatric disorder, treatment will depend on the diagnosis and other factors involved. The patient may be found to have a depressive disorder, in which case he will have to be treated accordingly (e.g. antidepressants, cognitive/behavioural/psychodynamic psychotherapy). However, it must be taken into account that most psychotropic drugs can cause impotence. If he has functional impotence and anxiety symptoms in the presence of marital disharmony, marital therapy would be appropriate. Marital distress and sexual dysfunction are closely related. In a recent study, a significant proportion of couples referred to a sexual dysfunction clinic were found to have psychiatric disorders. More than one-third were found to have marital problems. The patient should be persuaded to bring his wife for assessment and treatment of both as a couple. Alternatively, they could be referred for guidance to an agency such as Relate. Marital therapy should be offered. Behavioural, analytic or transactional methods can be used.

If appropriate, the couple can be referred to a sexual dysfunction clinic at a later stage, where their suitability for treatment will be assessed. The Masters and Johnson technique of 'sensate focus' and its variations have proved to be helpful for couples who are able to complete the treatment. Steps involved in sex therapy include relaxation exercises and systematic desensitisation ('homework'). Intracavernosal injection of vasoactive agents (e.g. papaverine/phentolamine) seems to be helpful in the management of impotence, and assessment for this treatment could be considered.

FURTHER READING

Bodner D R 1985 Impotence: evaluation and treatment. Primary Care 12(4): 719–733

Catalan J, Hawton K E, Day A 1990 Couples referred to a sexual dysfunction clinic. Psychological and physical morbidity. British Journal of Psychiatry 156: 61–67

Hawton K E 1989 Sexual disorders. Current Opinion in Psychiatry 2: 244–247

Rust J, Golombok S, Collier J 1988 Marital problems and sexual dysfunction: how are they related? British Journal of Psychiatry 152: 629–631

Szasz G, Stevenson R W, Lee L, Sanders H D 1987 Induction of penile erection by intracavernosal injection: a double blind comparison of phenoxybenzamine versus papaverine-phentolamine versus saline. Archives of Sexual Behaviour 16(5): 371–378

A18

A heroin addict presents to the accident and emergency department feeling depressed and physically unwell

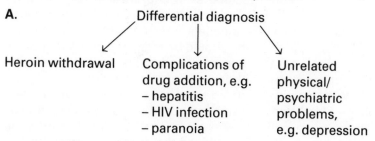

A.   Differential diagnosis

Heroin withdrawal   Complications of drug addition, e.g.
– hepatitis
– HIV infection
– paranoia

Unrelated physical/psychiatric problems, e.g. depression

B. Management of heroin withdrawal:

– detoxification
– withdrawal agents: methadone, clonidine
– associated treatments (e.g. therapeutic groups)
– rehabilitation

Depression in a 28-year-old heroin addict may or may not be related to the fact that he is drug-dependent. Likely reasons for his attending are that he wants help to withdraw from heroin, that he is unable to obtain his supply of the drugs and has fears of withdrawal symptoms, or that he has some complications from his drug addiction. The full assessment will include a physical as well as a psychiatric examination. It is important to obtain detailed information about the source of his drugs and the method of administration, e.g. sharing needles. Information should also be obtained about symptoms suggestive of serious complications of drug use, e.g. HIV infection (weight loss, fatigue, repeated infections, swellings or ulcers and neurological impairment). Symptoms of opiate withdrawal would include irritability, lacrimation, abdominal cramps, gooseflesh, yawning and insomnia. Other details of importance are his social circumstances, previous psychiatric history, forensic history and current financial circumstances. Careful physical examination should be carried out to establish any of the physical complications that could occur as a result of chronic intravenous drug administration. Mental state examination may reveal evidence of cognitive impairment in association with his depression. The severity of his depression should be assessed. Further investigations would include screening for hepatitis B and, if necessary, with his consent and after counselling, for HIV infection. Other investigations could include skull and chest X-ray and a CT scan. The presence of serious physical illness or psychiatric illness would call for inpatient management. In the absence of any complication, he should be managed on an outpatient basis. Treatment should be aimed at his current presenting symptoms, heroin withdrawal and rehabilitation.

Withdrawing opiate addicts from drugs is the preliminary stage of treatment. Methadone can be used as a withdrawal agent, given orally as a syrup. It can be administered in an initial dose from 20–70 mg, and the dosage progressively reduced until detoxification is completed. Clonidine can also be used. The detoxification programme should be accompanied by activities such as therapeutic groups, community meetings and individual counselling, which should aim at motivating the patients to complete the treatment and ensuring compliance. Long-term rehabilitation must be planned at the beginning of withdrawal.

If it proves difficult to initiate a withdrawal regime using methadone, it would be appropriate to admit the patient for a brief period of up to one week in order to assess the amount of methadone that he would need to replace his current intake of heroin. If withdrawal is not possible, a maintenance programme with methadone should be instituted. This would prevent the patient from seeking supplies of drugs on the street, and give him a reason for staying in contact with the drug dependence clinic. Advice on the risks of HIV infection should be given. Aftercare should include contact with a drug dependence unit, a community drug team or an outpatient clinic. Rehabilitation should aim to remove the patient from the drug culture and to give him the opportunity to develop new social contacts. He should also be put in touch with self-help groups such as Narcotics Anonymous (NA).

FURTHER READING

Evans D L, Perkins D O 1990 The clinical psychiatry of AIDS. Current Opinion in Psychiatry 3: 96–102

Ghodse A H, London M, Bewley T H, Bhat A V 1987 Inpatient treatment for drug abuse. British Journal of Psychiatry 151: 72–75

Gossop M, Griffiths P, Bradley B, Strang J 1989 Opiate withdrawal symptoms in response to 10-day and 21-day methadone withdrawal programmes. British Journal of Psychiatry 154: 360–363

London M, Ghodse A H 1989 Types of opiate addiction and notification to the home office. British Journal of Psychiatry 154: 835–838

A19

This boy has made a serious attempt at suicide. In the assessment, one should get as detailed an account as is possible from him about the incident and his understanding of the consequences of his act. Does he wish he was dead? What are the reasons for his truanting from school? How does he perceive himself at school and at home? His recent problems at school may be related to serious problems such as severe bullying and sexual abuse, or due to his inability to cope with the curriculum. He may be finding it difficult to live up to his family's academic expectations of him. His thoughts and feelings about these issues should be tactfully explored. Admission may be necessary for a full assessment, as this may not be possible in the accident and emergency department.

The boy's mother should be seen on her own to assess the family situation, particularly the attitude of both parents and other significant relatives to the child's problems at school, and their reaction to his attempt at suicide. It is important to obtain a complete family history, especially that of psychiatric illness, suicide, family conflict and physical or sexual abuse.

If the boy needs to be observed for physical reasons, he should be admitted to a paediatric ward, and treatment of the physical state takes priority. If the child is felt to be in danger of repeating the attempt, or if his safety is felt to be compromised in any way, he should be treated as an inpatient, regardless of his physical state. If the parents refuse permission, a place of safety order should be applied for. Even in the absence of any reasons necessitating hospital admission, a short admission on a paediatric ward may be advisable, in order to facilitate a complete psychiatric and social evaluation. The child also need not return immediately to a highly charged family environment that could be hostile. A complete assessment should be done by the child psychiatric team within a couple of days, and the child discharged unless there are indications for a longer hospital stay, such as severe depression, or if there are doubts about his safety if he returns home. If this is the case, he should be transferred to a child psychiatric unit. However, keeping in mind the history of problems at school and at home, and his age, it is unlikely that a depressive illness has led to the attempt.

The problems at school should be addressed, the boy's teacher and educational psychologist involved in the management, and an early return to school facilitated. The family doctor should be notified and involved. The parents should be helped to deal with their anxiety about the situation, and educated about measures they should take to prevent any further attempts at self-harm by their son. These include responding effectively to their child when he is in trouble, being more realistic in their expectations of him, taking adequate practical measures such as locking the medicine cabinet, etc. Further treatment could include individual psychotherapy or counselling for the child, and family and marital therapy or counselling. An expert social worker should be involved in the long-term treatment. Careful follow-up is essential, as there is a significant risk of repetition. Follow-up could be effectively done by the family practitioner and the social worker, with the help of the child psychiatric team if necessary.

FURTHER READING

Black M, Erulkar J, Kerfoot M, Meadow R, Baderman H 1982 The management of parasuicide in young people under sixteen. The Bulletin of The Royal College of Psychiatrists 6: 182–185

Brooksbank D J 1985 Suicide and parasuicide in childhood and early adolescence. British Journal of Psychiatry 146: 459–463

Shaffer D 1974 Suicide in childhood and early adolescence. Journal of Child Psychology and Psychiatry 15: 275–291

A20

The first step is to take a detailed history from the patient about the nature of his difficulties, bearing in mind the importance of obtaining an objective view from an informant. His current difficulty may be part of a longstanding psychiatric disorder, and a careful history would elucidate this. The history should also seek to elicit evidence of alcohol or drug abuse. A detailed mental state examination should be carried out to establish the precise nature of his belief system. His daughter should be interviewed to obtain her view of the problems as well as to get details of the onset and progression. She may be able to provide information on whether he has been acting on his beliefs by threatening the neighbours, being abusive to them or getting into fights with them. The persecutory ideas that he is expressing could be part of a functional disorder, or due to organic conditions, such as acute or chronic brain disorders, endocrine disorders, such as hyperparathyroidism, and drugs. A full physical examination combined with laboratory investigations will clarify the diagnosis.

The paranoid delusion may be part of a schizophrenic illness, in which case the patient will demonstrate other symptoms of schizophrenia. However, if there is no previous history, this would be fairly unusual because of its late onset. Manic-depressive illness, depressed type, could have paranoid symptoms as a major part of the presentation. In this case, there would be profound affective change consonant with the persecutory delusion.

The presence of an elaborate systematised delusion of persecution associated with reference, presenting at the age of 50 years in the absence of other psychopathology, would suggest a diagnosis of paranoid state. There is much controversy about the validity of this separate category, despite the fact that it exists in both ICD-9 and DSM-III. Some authors suggest that it should be considered late-onset, better prognosis, schizophrenia.

The decision to admit will be strongly influenced by the daughter's and any other report of aggressive or dangerous consequences of his beliefs, e.g. threatening the neighbours, attacking them or getting involved with useless visits to the police or lawyers. Compulsory admission may be necessary. Every effort should be made to preserve a good therapeutic relationship without colluding with the patients beliefs. Underlying physical problems should be treated. A suitable neuroleptic drug may relieve the symptoms. Psychological support and encouragement should also be offered. Support should also be offered to the daughter, as she will play a major role in his continuing care.

FURTHER READING

Munro A 1988 Delusional (paranoid) disorder: etiologic and taxonomic considerations: II A possible relationship between delusional and affective disorders. Canadian Journal of Psychiatry 33: 171–174

A21

A problem of this description presenting soon after a tragic event such as the Bradford football stadium disaster could be post-traumatic stress disorder (PTSD). However, other possibilities should be considered, such as:

– anxiety state unrelated to a specific acute traumatic event
– situational crises
– depressive illness
– organic condition, e.g. temporal lobe epilepsy.

A detailed history from the patient and any other informants, as well as careful examination of his mental state, will help to clarify the diagnosis.

With complex partial seizures or temporal lobe epilepsy (TLE), there is commonly a history of birth injury, anoxia or febrile convulsions in infancy. His repeated 'dreaming' could be depersonalisation, déja vu and dreamlike reminiscence which occur in complex partial seizures, so a very careful account should be taken of when they occur, the nature of these experiences and whether they are accompanied by the smell of burning, which may be an olfactory hallucination. Other features of complex partial seizures which should be explored are the 'epigastric aura', and autonomic effects, such as salivation and flushing. Strong feelings of fear and anxiety may be part of the aura, and witnesses may have noticed characteristic movements of his lips and mouth as if he were chewing, tasting or swallowing. The diagnosis may be confirmed by an abnormal electroencephalogram (EEG). A sleep EEG, and EEG done with sphenoidal leads may be necessary before abnormalities are detected. Failure to detect EEG changes does not exclude a diagnosis of complex partial seizures, as this is a clinical diagnosis. The first line of treatment of this condition is carbamazepine.

The criteria for diagnosing PTSD as described by the DSM-III-R include:

- The experience of an unusual event which would be extremely distressing for almost anyone. This experience is associated with intense fear, terror and helplessness.
- Re-experience of the traumatic event which may take the form of vivid dreams, illusions and hallucinations, as well as episodes of 'flashback'.
- Reminders of the trauma may be associated with intense psychological distress.
- Avoidance of stimuli associated with the trauma.
- Sleep difficulties, irritability, difficulty in concentration and general hyperarousal.

The diagnosis of PTSD is usually made after the symptoms have been present for at least a month, although symptoms could start years after the disaster.

The primary aetiological factor in the development of this condition has been thought to be the nature and the extent of the stress. However, a recent study suggests that neither the degree of exposure to stress nor the losses sustained were as good predictors of PTSD as were neuroticism or past history of psychological treatment.

Treatment options include: dynamic psychotherapy with abreaction, reconstruction of the traumatic event and replication of the experience and behavioural-cognitive treatment which concentrates on the causes of the stress, the failed coping mechanisms already used and ways of optimising coping mechanisms. Pharmacological intervention may also be beneficial for alleviation of distressing symptoms.

In this particular case, a definite treatment plan can only be determined after all the information is elicited.

FURTHER READING

Bleich A, Garb R, Kottler M 1986 Treatment of prolonged combat reaction. British Journal of Psychiatry 148: 493–496

Burges Watson I P, Hoffman L, Wilson G V 1988 The neuropsychiatry of
    post-traumatic stress disorder. British Journal of Psychiatry 152: 164–173

Daly D D 1975 Ictal clinical manifestations of complex partial seizures. In:
    Penry J K, Daly D (eds) Advances in neurology Vol II. Raven Press, New
    York

McFarlane A C 1989 The aetiology of post-traumatic morbidity:
    predisposing, precipitating and perpetuating factors. British Journal of
    Psychiatry 154: 221–228

Reynolds E H, Trimble M R 1981 Epilepsy and psychiatry. Churchill
    Livingstone, Edinburgh

A22

One would offer her an outpatient appointment, to which she
should be invited to bring her spouse, partner or a close relative. Before seeing the patient, it would be wise to talk to her
general practitioner over the telephone, in order to obtain any
further information that one may find necessary.

When she is seen, the following points should be covered
in the assessment:

1. The exact nature and duration of the patient's depression. Is the patient mildly depressed all the time with
occasional exacerbations, or does she feel normal between
episodes of depression? When she is at her worst, does she
have symptoms such as general anhedonia, retardation, biological features such as loss of appetite, severe guilt, depressive delusions, reduced libido, altered sleep, feelings of
hopelessness and suicidal ideas? If so, she is likely to have a
major depressive illness. However, a 10-year history of mild
depression that has been managed mainly by her general
practitioner makes this unlikely. Persistence of affective
symptoms, however mild, and/or impaired social functioning
as a result would suggest chronic depression or a depressive
personality. Symptoms of mild depression include a feeling
of sadness, low self-esteem, tearfulness, loss of energy,
anxiety, poor concentration and increased or decreased sleep
and appetite. Whatever the severity of her depression, it
could be *secondary* to a physical illness (e.g. rheumatoid
arthritis, hypothyroidism), any medication she may be taking,
or another psychiatric problem, and it is essential that such

causative factors are identified. Anxiety and other neurotic disorders are sometimes mistakenly labelled as depression, and these should be looked for. Inadequately treated episodes of major depression can lead to a state of chronic depression, so it is important to obtain all details of any treatment she may have had in the past.

2. Predisposing and precipitating factors. These would include factors such as loss or separation from parents in childhood, an unhappy or traumatic childhood (e.g. sexual abuse), chronic stress (marital/sexual problems, general dissatisfaction with life, the frustrations of being a teacher, caring for a disabled person, etc.), lack of any social support, premenstrual mood changes, recent life events, family history of an affective or other psychiatric disorder.

3. The effects of her depression on her personal life. Has she had difficulty in making and keeping relationships or jobs? Has she resorted to excessive alcohol use? How have her friends and relatives responded to her depression? Has her social life suffered?

Recommendations for treatment would depend on the nature and severity and of her depression.

For example, if she had an unhappy childhood, with loss or rejection, along with low self-esteem and a poor ability to make and keep relationships, individual insight-oriented psychotherapy would be indicated. This could help her gain insight into her problem, improve her self-esteem, enable her to deal with intimate relationships, losses, etc. Cognitive therapy would be indicated if she is someone who has a very negative concept of herself, of her future and of the outside world. Depression in these circumstances is thought to be a result of the person's negative attitudes. Treatment is carried out in 12 weekly sessions, in which she will be helped to identify and test negative cognitions, and to develop and rehearse alternative, more positive ways of thinking. If her social functioning is impaired in the setting of mild depression, she may benefit from group therapy. Interpersonal therapy, which is currently used mainly in the United States, could also help, but it is unlikely to be available easily in the United Kingdom. This consists of 12 to 16 weekly sessions, in which issues such as lack of assertiveness or poor social skills are addressed, *only* in the context of their meaning or effect on interpersonal relationships. The choice of psychotherapy would also depend on the availability of, and on her attitude to psychotherapy. Her general practitioner may be able to offer her supportive psychotherapy at his practice, and unravel situational and personality problems, once you have ruled out a major affective illness or an underlying primary problem.

If the patient has a major affective disorder, appropriate pharmacotherapy, in the form of antidepressants or lithium, should be commenced. If the depression is not severe, but all the same chronic and disabling, with atypical features, a course of monoamine oxidase inhibitors may be beneficial.

Any consequences of her depression should also be addressed. For example, there may be marital problems, and either counselling or marital therapy may be indicated. Her depression should be discussed with her immediate family and any appropriate support given.

One would write back to the general practitioner with a summary of the assessment and the recommendations, and make the appropriate psychotherapy referrals, if necessary. Further follow-up can be offered by the general practitioner, unless there is a specific indication for psychiatric follow-up.

FURTHER READING

Dobson K S 1989 A meta-analysis of the efficacy of cognitive therapy for depression. Journal of Consulting and Clinical Psychology 57: 414–419

Fennell M J V, Frances J A 1987 Cognitive therapy for depression: individual differences and the process of change. Cognitive Therapy Research 11: 253–271

Klerman G L, Weissman M M, Rounsaville B J, Chevron R S (eds) 1984 Interpersonal psychotherapy of depression. Basic Books, New York

Paykel E S 1989 Treatment of depression: the relevance of research for clinical practice. British Journal of Psychiatry 155: 754–763

Scott J 1988 Chronic depression. British Journal of Psychiatry 153: 287–297

A23

15-year-old girl, behavioural problems and decline in performance after recent bereavement

A.

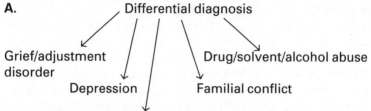

Differential diagnosis

Grief/adjustment disorder

Depression

Drug/solvent/alcohol abuse

Familial conflict

Early schizophrenia/manic-depressive illness

B. Assessment (multidisciplinary/involve family)

- Previous adjustment and level of functioning
- Family conflicts
- Role of grandmother/effect of her death on patient/family
- Parental illness/marital conflict

- Problems at school
- Peer group relationships
- Sexual adjustment/ problems
- Abuse of psychoactive agents
- Physical examination
- Mental state examination

C. Treatment

- Is treatment necessary?
- Who should be treated (patient/family/both)?
- What treatment is indicated and practicable?

Treatment options (one or more of the following):
- Grief counselling for individual/family
- Individual psychotherapy/family therapy
- Treat psychiatric/physical illness if present.

Onset of behavioural problems along with poor performance at school, at the age of 15, following the death of her grandmother, suggests a bereavement reaction. Often, familial problems tend to surface, or become more prominent after a bereavement, and this could be another reason for the change in the patient's behaviour. She could have started using drugs during this period of stress, or be experiencing difficulties in her relationships with her peers or with sexual adjustment. Early schizophrenia or manic depressive illness, though uncommon at this age, could have been precipitated or accelerated by the death, and may present with these problems.

The assessment, outlined in the flow diagram, should cover all these possibilities. The patient's behavioural changes may be an entirely normal reaction to her grandmother's death. The only intervention that may be required is explanation and reassurance. If, on the other hand, she is still grieving over the loss of her grandmother, 3 months after her death, she should be helped to come to terms with the death. Individual sessions in which she is encouraged to talk and reminisce about her grandmother, express her feelings about her (whether positive or negative), and her fears about how the death will change life for her, may help. If the family has found the death difficult to cope with, they could benefit from grief counselling. The school should be involved, and given guidance about how to deal with the situation. Any other problems that are revealed during the assessment should be dealt with. The patient should be followed up carefully, as these symptoms could indicate continuing behavioural and personality problems, or the development of schizophrenia or manic-depressive illness at a later age.

FURTHER READING

Van Eerdewegh M M, Clayton P J, Eerdewegh P 1985 The bereaved child: variables influencing early psychopathology. British Journal of Psychiatry 147: 188–194

A24

A. Behavioural disturbance in a patient remanded in custody

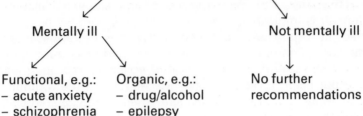

Mentally ill		Not mentally ill
Functional, e.g.: – acute anxiety – schizophrenia	Organic, e.g.: – drug/alcohol – epilepsy	No further recommendations

B.   Appropriate treatment

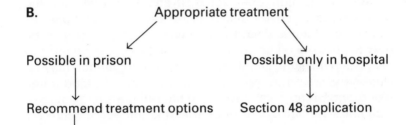

Possible in prison	Possible only in hospital
Recommend treatment options	Section 48 application

No further action UNLESS court requests report later

The assessment will be aimed at elucidating whether the man's 'bizarre' behaviour is, in fact, a result of physical or psychiatric problems, so that appropriate treatment can be given. A person can be held on remand, waiting to appear before a magistrates court or a crown court, and it is important to know which court is involved.

One should get a careful account, from more than one staff member who was present, about the circumstances under which the 'bizarre' behaviour started, the temporal progression and a detailed description. Being disinhibited, aggressive, vague and inaccessible, posturing, or responding to auditory hallucinations are all examples of what could be termed 'bizarre' behaviour, and each of these points to different underlying problems. It is vital to know the interval between the onset of the problem and his being taken into custody, and his condition when taken into custody. A short interval (few days) and no remarkable features when taken into custody points to a drug or alcohol withdrawal-induced state, particularly if the theft was committed in order to obtain money. Being a stockbroker, he may be in a stressful job and vulnerable to drug and alcohol abuse. Stresses may also derive from personal circumstances at home and in his relationships. It is important to enquire in detail about his previous medical history and treatment, and it may be necessary to contact his general practitioner for these details. An important differential diagnosis is that of epilepsy, and one must ask specifically if the staff have noticed any features pointing to epilepsy (pre-ictal and post-ictal phenomena, altered consciousness, convulsions, etc.).

After evaluation, one should be able to say whether the person's disturbed behaviour is related to a functional or organic psychiatric disorder, and what treatment should be offered. The prison doctor may be able to treat the person in the prison hospital, and if so, no further intervention may be necessary after making recommendations for appropriate treatment. Urgent treatment could be necessary in a hospital. If so, the psychiatrist can recommend to the Home Secretary that the prisoner be transferred to a hospital, under Section 48 of the Mental Health Act 1983, which can only be used for mental illness and severe mental impairment. Another medical practitioner will have to support this recommendation (one of the practitioners should be approved under Section 12). The Home Secretary will have to consider the transfer expedient, a hospital should be willing to accept the patient and the patient should be moved within 14 days of the transfer direction. The courts are not involved, and the prison doctor can contact a local consultant psychiatrist directly, as in this case, to expedite the whole procedure. The patient can stay in hospital until he is able to return to prison and continue the remand. If he is on remand by the crown court, the date of appearance at the crown court can be altered. If on remand by a magistrates court, he can be detained only for the length of his remand. However, the court can renew the remand to allow him to continue in hospital until fully treated.

If he does not improve, and it appears that he is unlikely to be fit for the trial, the transfer direction can be converted to a hospital order (Section 37). The conversion can be made by the court, in the absence of the prisoner and without a conviction, on the basis of oral or written evidence given by two doctors, provided all the conditions for a hospital order are fulfilled.

A25

The most likely diagnosis in this case is acute porphyria. The diagnosis may be substantiated by a positive family history, although this may not be elicited because inheritance is by an autosomal dominant gene with incomplete penetrance.

Other clinical features which may be present are pain in the limbs and back, headache, weakness and numbness of the limbs and peripheral neuropathy. The mental state may fluctuate between violence and depression, and may include psychotic phenomena resembling schizophrenia and paranoid reactions.

The violence is best managed by promazine 100–200 mg intramuscularly. Chlorpromazine and trifluoperazine can also be given. Barbiturates are likely to aggravate the attack and are contraindicated, as are thioridazine and zuclopenthixol hydrochloride (Clopixol).

The precipitants of acute attacks of porphyria include acute infection, alcohol and various other drugs. Any infection should be treated immediately, but sulphonamides, griseofulvin and chloroquine should be avoided as they worsen attacks. Other drugs to avoid are dichloralphenalzone (Welldorm), methyldopa and thiopentone. Should the patient require ECT, it will have to be given without an anaesthetic to avoid precipitating paralysis and respiratory failure. It would be advisable for an anaesthetist to be present during ECT. The patient's level of hydration should be monitored, because the persistent vomiting may induce electrolyte imbalance.

About 20% of cases develop epileptic seizures which may progress to status epilepticus. The ward staff must be warned against the dangers of using barbiturates and advised to use paraldehyde instead.

FURTHER READING

Goldberg A, Moore M R, McColl K E L, Brodie M J 1987 Porphyrin metabolism and the porphyrias. In: Oxford Textbook of Medicine Vol. 1, 2nd edn: (eds) Weatherall D J, Ledingham J G G, Warrell D A Oxford University Press, Oxford

A26

A 3-year-old boy with behavioural and communication problems

A. Differential diagnosis

Deafness   Severe   Mental   Genetic   Infantile
            deprivation   retardation   disorders   autism

B. Assessment:

– Birth: pregnancy (e.g. alcohol, intrauterine infection)
           delivery (e.g. anoxia, complications)
           metabolic disorders (e.g. phenylketonuria)
– Developmental history: motor, language and social
                           milestone, e.g.
                           deafness
                           low IQ
                           infantile autism
– Family history: e.g.   genetic/psychiatric disorder
                         social/financial problems
– Examination: communication skills (speech/
                 comprehension)
                 social overtures/responses/play
                 IQ/level of development
                 physical/neurological status
– Investigations for: e.g.   chromosomal abnormalities
                             sexually transmitted diseases
                             porphyria/mucopolysaccharidosis.

C. Further management:

– Audiological and visual tests
– Specialised assessment and treatment
– Social services
– Help to the family (e.g. financial, at home)
– Multidisciplinary team (e.g. speech/behavioural therapist)
– Special education

This is a 3-year-old child with behavioural and communication difficulties. Possible causes of his problems include deafness, severe forms of deprivation, mental retardation, genetic
disorders or a pervasive developmental disorder (e.g. infan-

tile autism). A clear account of the nature of his problems should be obtained from his parents, including aspects such as language (e.g. expression, comprehension), behaviour (e.g. playing, occupation) and social interaction (e.g. attachments, social responses). It is essential to know when his problems began, especially whether or not they were preceded by a period of normal development. In addition, his present level of development must be investigated.

In taking his history, problems during pregnancy, such as heavy smoking, use of drugs (e.g. anti-epileptics) and alcohol consumption by the mother, or the occurrence of intrauterine infection (e.g. cytomegalovirus) should be looked for. Circumstances of birth, such as premature delivery, anoxia, low birth weight or complications at delivery must be explored. Jaundice or a metabolic disorder (e.g. phenylketonuria) may have been detected. If so, it is important to know how this was dealt with. The child may have had a physical illness, such as meningitis or encephalitis. His developmental history must be assessed in detail, covering motor (e.g. sitting, crawling, standing, walking), language (e.g. babbling, 'dada' or 'mama', imitating sounds, words) and social (e.g. smiling responsively/spontaneously, reaction to parents/strangers, imitating, playing) milestones. Hearing loss should be considered if the child does not respond to ordinary household sounds. Information on his family situation must be obtained (e.g. social and financial difficulties, psychiatric problems). A history of parental neglect or abuse may be present. However, a history of general failure to develop social relationships (e.g. no selective attachment, no group playing), language retardation (e.g. impaired babbling, no gain of useful speech) with impaired comprehension, and stereotypical behaviour and routines (e.g. flapping of hands, pirouetting) with onset *before* 30 months would lead to the diagnosis of infantile autism. If this seems to be the case, the presence of other underlying handicaps (e.g. low IQ) should be explored.

The examination must cover his communication skills (e.g. speech, comprehension), his social overtures (e.g. visual gaze, facial expressions) and social responses (e.g. eye-to-eye contact, reciprocity). His social play (e.g. spontaneous imitation, humour, co-operation), his playing with toys (e.g. repetitive and/or ritualistic play) and how he keeps himself occupied (e.g. playing with his fingers, spinning, doing nothing) are aspects which also should be observed. The physical and neurological examination must include the measurement of his head circumference, weight and height. Further investigations would include screening for chromosomal, metabolic and endocrine abnormalities.

Further management will be determined by the findings of the assessment. For example, if the child is suspected to be deaf, sophisticated audiological tests may prove necessary. The involvement of social services is essential if evidence of deprivation is detected. If he is diagnosed as having infantile autism, management will depend on factors such as his level of development (language, behaviour, social) and IQ. This should aim to foster his development and learning, to reduce stereotypies and maladaptive behaviour (e.g. tantrums) and to help the family. A multidisciplinary team approach (e.g. psychologist, speech therapist, behavioural therapist, social worker) is fundamental. The diagnosis of infantile autism and its implications (e.g. handicaps, prognosis) should be carefully explained to the parents. A programme to teach spoken or non-vocal (signing) language would be appropriate. Techniques to promote learning, such as chaining or prompt finding, could be helpful. Engagement in play should be encouraged, and behavioural methods (e.g. to reduce stereotypies/maladaptive behaviour) can prove most useful. The parents should participate as co-therapists. Practical help such as baby sitting, holiday provisions and financial allowances should be available. Provisions for special education must be planned in advance. Agencies such as the National Autistic Society can prove invaluable (e.g. advice on education, special schools).

FURTHER READING

Goodman R 1989 Infantile autism: a syndrome of multiple primary deficits? Journal of Autism and Developmental Disorders 19(3): 409–424

Levitas A 1990 Developmental and family aspects of autism. Pediatric Annals 19(1): 52–58

Rutter M 1985 Infantile autism and other pervasive developmental disorders. In: Rutter M, Hersov L Child and adolescent psychiatry: modern approaches. Blackwell Scientific, London, pp 545–566

Volkmar F R, Cohen D J 1989 Disintegrative disorder or 'late onset' autism. Journal of Child Psychology and Psychiatry and Allied Disciplines 30(5): 717–724

A27

This is a woman with a mental illness related to the puerperium. Onset within 2 weeks of delivery would suggest puerperal psychosis, and the history and examination would be seeking to support or refute this. When taking the history, particular attention should be given to any family history of schizophrenia or manic-depressive illness. Other important predisposing and precipitating factors to establish are marital problems, lack of family or other social support, unplanned pregnancy, difficulties during the pregnancy and birth, and difficulties with the child. Puerperal psychosis is more likely to occur in primiparous women than in multiparous women. Examination of the patient may reveal clouding of consciousness. The majority of puerperal psychoses are manic in nature, but careful examination should be carried out to establish the exact nature of the psychosis in this patient, as this will determine treatment. This patient appears to have both affective and schizophreniform symptoms, a picture not uncommon in puerperal psychosis. There is usually marked fluctuation in the severity and the type of symptoms. It is possible that she has an organic psychosis. Careful examination of her physical as well as her mental state is essential. Particular attention should be given to ideas of self harm or of harm to the baby. It is vital to establish what her feelings are towards the baby and whether she has any abnormal beliefs about the baby. Both depressed and schizophrenic patients may have beliefs that their children are abnormal or evil, and this may lead to attempts to kill them.

Given the nature of her symptoms, arrangements should be made to admit the patient and the baby to a specialised mother-and-baby unit. If she refuses admission to hospital, she may have to be compulsorily admitted if there is risk to herself or the baby. Treatment should be commenced with a suitable neuroleptic, such as haloperidol or chlorpromazine. Secretion does occur through breast milk, but in very small quantities and there is no evidence of detrimental effects on infants. If there is no improvement within four weeks, electroconvulsive therapy, which is particularly useful in this condition, is usually commenced. Additionally, there should be good nursing care with supervised care of the baby. As the patient improves, she should take increasing responsibility for the baby. The husband should be involved in the care as much as possible. Some mother and baby units have facilities for fathers to sleep in, and share in the care of the new baby. Prior to discharge, careful assessment of the mother's ability to care for the child independently has to be carried out. Discharge will depend on her improved mental state, and her ability to care for the baby, as well as the level of support that she is likely to have at home. Most patients recover or improve within 3 months, but about one-third of those who become pregnant again will have a recurrence. About 40% of women who have a puerperal psychosis will have a further psychotic episode. The patient and the family should be advised of the risk of recurrence, as should the general practitioner.

FURTHER READING

Brockington I F, Kumar R 1982 Motherhood and mental illness. Academic Press, London

Meltzer E S, Kumar R 1985 Puerperal mental illness, clinical features and classification: a study of 142 mother-and-baby admissions. British Journal of Psychiatry 147: 647–654

Platz C, Kendell R E 1988 A matched-control follow-up and family study of 'puerperal psychoses'. British Journal of Psychiatry 153: 90–94

A28

This man may be suffering from anxiety or depression, or a combination of these. As he has an unsettled claim for compensation he is likely to have a 'compensation neurosis'. The prolonged nature of his symptoms and the antecedent events would suggest that the aetiological factors are psychological rather than organic. In the early stages of 'post-concussional syndrome' the symptoms are more likely to be of organic origin. However, these recede with time. The prolongation of symptoms may be related to factors unrelated to the accident, such as psychosocial difficulties pre-dating the accident; life events immediately before the accident; and longstanding personality difficulties. It will be important to get a detailed social, occupational, marital and sexual history in order to obtain a baseline from which deviations subsequent to the accident can be observed. A detailed account of the circumstances of the accident, and the patient's emotional response at the time should be obtained, as they may be contributing to the prolongation of the symptoms. The symptoms he experienced immediately after the road traffic accident should be ascertained, as well as the explanation he received for them. If he were given inadequate explanations for his symptoms, whilst at the same time was subjected to repeated and extensive investigations, this may have contributed to the long-term nature of his difficulties. Financial, relationship or other psycho-social difficulties he experienced since the accident, as well the idea of pursuing compensation, would probably play a major part in this man's chronic difficulties. Financial compensation does not necessarily mean that his difficulties will resolve, nor will lack of compensation necessarily prevent resolution. Given the prolonged nature of his symptoms, he may well remain chronically disabled.

FURTHER READING

Kelly R, Smith B N 1981 Post-traumatic syndrome: another myth discredited. Journal of the Royal Society of Medicine 79: 275–277

Lishman W A 1973 The psychiatric sequelae of head injury: a review. Psychological Medicine 3: 304–318

Lishman W A 1988 Physiogenesis and psychogenesis in the 'post-concussional syndrome'. British Journal of Psychiatry 153: 460–469

Tarsh M J, Royston C 1985 A follow-up study of accident neurosis. British Journal of Psychiatry 146: 18–25

A29

Although it is clear that affective disorders tend to cluster in families, and that genetic factors are involved in their aetiology, studies on affective disorders often present different results because of different diagnostic criteria. Genetic influence is more evident in severe affective illness. However, what is inherited is not the certainty of becoming ill but, rather, a liability to develop the disorder. In the liability/threshold model, genes, environment or both may contribute. A single major locus, the polygenic/multifactorial model and the mixed model have all been postulated as a genetic hypothesis for affective disorder.

If a classification of endogenous (bipolar/unipolar) versus non-endogenous is adopted, lifetime morbid risk in the general population for endogenous affective disorder is about 2.6% (under 1% for bipolar and about 3% for unipolar disorder), and ranges from 3 to 9% for non-endogenous affective disorder. Conversely, risk for first-degree relatives ranges from 15 to 20%, and from 10 to 15% for bipolar and unipolar disorders respectively, whereas family incidence of non-endogenous depression is lower.

Information on the woman's mother's psychiatric history must be obtained. It must be confirmed whether she has, in fact, an affective illness, or suffers from another psychiatric condition. Any other family history of psychiatric illness, on both the mother's and the father's sides, should be investigated.

If her mother had a bipolar disorder, the risk of an affective disorder for the client, either unipolar or bipolar, will be greater than that for the general population. On the other hand, if her mother had a 'neurotic' depression, and the client has no psychiatric history or symptoms, her risk will be practically the same as that of the general population. The onset of a psychiatric condition will also depend on the presence of precipitating factors, such as stressful life experiences, and personality factors. It is important to explore whether her upbringing was affected by her mother's illness, and to what extent.

Risk for her children will depend on her and her fiancé's condition and family history. It will be highest if both have a bipolar disorder, and the same as that for the general population if neither is affected or has a family history. In any case, it would be worth discussing the woman's worries and doubts, and explaining that a history of affective illness in the family does not mean that this is necessarily going to be transmitted to the offspring. In fact, the probability of being affected is much lower than the probability of *not* being affected, and factors other than heredity also contribute to the development of mental illness.

FURTHER READING

Boyd J H, Weissman M M 1981 Epidemiology of affective disorders. Archives of General Psychiatry 38: 1039–1046

Merikangas K R, Weissman M M, Pauls D L 1985 Genetic factors in the sex ratio of major depression. Psychological Medicine 15: 63–69

McGuffin P, Katz R 1989 The genetics of depression and manic-depressive disorder. British Journal of Psychiatry 155: 294–304

Targum S D, Schulz S C 1982 Clinical application of psychiatric genetics. American Journal of Orthopsychiatry 52: 45–57

A30

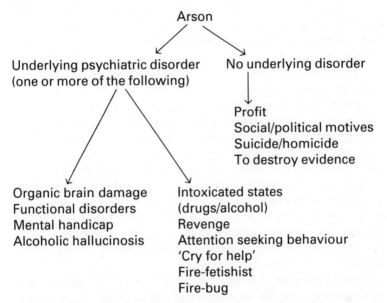

The aims of assessment are to establish whether there was a psychiatric disorder either at the time of the offence or since, and the motivation for the offence. Although the person is said to be mentally subnormal, there may be other reasons for the fire-setting behaviour and they should not be over-looked. More than one of the problems listed in the flow diagram may be operative at any one time. A 'fire bug' is a person in whom starting a fire seems to release tension. The fires are usually unplanned, and some individuals may start many fires within a short period. They are usually unplanned, and some individuals may start many fires within a short period. They are usually people with a background of person-ality disorder and poor social adjustment. 'Fire-fetishists' are people who gain overt sexual satisfaction from fire-raising. They are usually solitary people, and mental subnormality is more common in this group than in the general population.

If there is an underlying treatable problem such as schizo-phrenia, (e.g. fire-setting in response to auditory hallucina-tions), this condition has to be treated first. In this person, the presence of mental handicap and the history of previous offences implies that the risk of future arson episodes is con-siderable. This is particularly so if her fire-setting is precipi-tated by minor stress, and if there is evidence of persistent impulses to set fire. However, there is very little research evidence to guide psychiatrists in the accurate assessment of future dangerousness, and the courts should be made aware of this.

The report should cover the presence of psychiatric ab-normality, appropriate treatment and the best setting in which to offer it. If there is an underlying illness, treatment and rehabilitation should be the main aims, and not punish-ment; but her needs must always be balanced against those of the public, who could be endangered. If the risks of re-petition are considerable, and it is unsafe to treat her as an outpatient, in a psychiatric hospital or in a regional secure unit, or if admission to a special hospital is for some reason inappropriate, then treatment could be offered during a prison sentence at prison hospitals (e.g. Grendon Under-wood, which specialises in the treatment of arsonists). Treat-ment for arson where there is no underlying psychiatric disorder needs to be tailored to individual needs, and usually incorporates psychotherapy and behavioural techniques. Appropriate rehabilitation for this patient's mental handicap should also be mentioned. For example, she may be resorting to repeated arson in order to add some excitement to an otherwise dull life, or in order to get some attention, particu-larly since she is living on her own in the community, and may be lacking support and company. Improving her living conditions and offering adequate daytime and leisure activi-ties would make it unnecessary for her to resort to arson for the reasons mentioned above.

FURTHER READING

Faulk M 1979 Assessing dangerousness in firesetting. In: Hamilton J R, Freeman H (eds) Dangerousness: psychiatric assessment and management. Gaskell, London, pp 73–76

Lewis N D C, Yarnell H 1951 Pathological firesetting. Nervous and Mental Disease Monograph No 82, New York

Scott D 1978 The problems of malicious fire-raising. British Journal of
    Hospital Medicine 19: 259–263

Soothill K 1990 Arson. In: Bluglass R, Bowden P (eds) Principles and
    practice of forensic psychiatry. Churchill Livingstone, Edinburgh,
    pp 776–779

A31

A. The patient here has a major depressive episode with delusions and psychomotor retardation. He was treated with an
inadequate dose of dothiepin initially, but has also responded
poorly to an adequate dose of amitryptline. He has not improved and his life is suffering as a result.
ECT is indicated here for the following reasons:

- the nature of the depression; delusions with psychomotor
  retardation, which responds best to ECT and often poorly to
  antidepressants
- the need for rapid improvement; he has already been in
  hospital for three months and the personal consequences
  of his depression are quite major
- poor response to drug treatment, though this was on an inadequate dose in the case of dothiepin.

One should also ensure that an underlying physical illness
has been carefully investigated for. The procedure and complications of ECT should be explained to him and his family
and his consent obtained. If he is unable or unwilling to have
ECT, the treatment should be given under Section 3 of the
Mental Health Act 1983, and a second opinion from the
Mental Health Act Commissioners sought, under Section 58
of the Act.

B. No, this patient is unlikely to have resistant depression, as
he was treated inadequately. Although there is no universally
accepted definition of resistant depression, it generally indicates depression for which one or two antidepressant drugs
or ECT were given appropriately, but to no effect. In this instance, he may well respond to ECT.

If this patient did have resistant depression, then the first
step would be to review his diagnosis and to look for other
conditions that could have been missed. His non-response
may be due to the fact that he has an underlying illness such

as a malignancy or an endocrine dysfunction. He could be on anti-hypertensives or other drugs that could cause depression. The next step would be to review all the treatment that he has had so far. The adequacy of the dosage of drugs or of ECT (if given), and other factors that could affect drug response must be evaluated. These would include concurrent usage of other drugs that may interact with the antidepressants at the pharmacokinetic or the pharmacodynamic level (e.g. barbiturates induce liver enzymes and would cause more rapid metabolism of nortryptiline, leading to a drop in plasma levels). He may not be swallowing the antidepressant! Other factors that could be maintaining the depression despite treatment would include adverse psychosocial factors (marital problems, major problems in his business, etc).

If any of the above factors are unearthed, the optimal management would be to deal with them individually, while continuing with the general pharmacological and psychosocial principles of treatment. If no such factors are responsible for the continuing depression, then treatment needs to be modified. The first step would be to use an antidepressant with a different mode of action, for example change to a serotonergic antidepressant (fluvoxamine/fluoxetine) from a noradrenergic antidepressant (desipramine), or to a monoamine oxidase inhibitor from a tricyclic antidepressant. Alternatively, if there has been some response to the antidepressant in use, lithium and/or carbamazepine could be added to potentiate its effect. If the condition of the patient is such that a quick response to treatment is needed, as in the patient in question, then ECT should be given. It must be emphasised that, however 'heroic' the physical treatment of resistant depression, the general principles of psychological treatment of depression should not be overlooked.

FURTHER READING

Nierenberg A A, Amsterdam M D 1990 Treatment of resistant depression; definition and treatment approaches. Journal of Clinical Psychiatry 51(6; suppl): 39–47

Hamilton M 1986 Electroconvulsive therapy: indications and contraindications. Annals of the New York Academy of Sciences 462: 5–11

Kendell R E 1981 The present status of electroconvulsive therapy. British Journal of Psychiatry 149: 265–383

A32

A 22-year-old girl seeking nose reconstruction

Underlying psychiatric condition   No psychiatric disorder

Organic, e.g.:   Functional, e.g.;
– epilepsy   – depression
– intracranial tumour   – schizophrenia
                            – monosymptomatic
                              delusional disorder

Treatment of underlying disorder: Advice to the
– antidepressants   plastic surgeon
– antipsychotics
– behavioural

This is a girl who seems to be disproportionately worried about a minor defect on her nose. The assessment should clarify whether or not this is a part of a psychiatric disorder, and what risks and benefits cosmetic surgery would entail.

Details of her personal history, personality and social circumstances must be obtained. Since her complaint started after her boyfriend left, she may have an underlying depressive disorder, in which case other symptoms, such as a poor self-image, low self-esteem, depressive feelings, loss of appetite and sleep disturbance, may also be present. Disturbance of body image may also occur in obsessive-compulsive disorder, schizophrenia and personality disorder. Dysmorphophobia is a persistent complaint of a specific bodily defect that is not noticeable to others, which occurs in the absence of any other psychiatric symptoms.

The advice given to this girl will depend firstly on whether or not there is a psychiatric condition. Inpatient treatment may be indicated if she is severely socially and/or functionally disabled by her problems. If a depressive disorder is diagnosed, treatment would involve antidepressants, support and counselling and psychotherapy (cognitive, behavioural or insight-orientated therapy). If she has schizophrenia, treatment will include neuroleptics, support and counselling and rehabilitation. For monosymptomatic delusional disorder, treatment with neuroleptics may be beneficial. Pimozide is said to be particularly effective in this condition, but there is some controversy over this claim. Moreover, a thorough physical evaluation is essential before pimozide is prescribed, given the association between the use of this drug and sudden unexpected death, even in young people. Psychodynamic psychotherapy or behavioural methods, such as desensitisation, assertiveness training and exposure therapy, may also be beneficial. These complaints might be the first indication of a serious functional illness (e.g. schizophrenia) and, in this case, this patient should be followed up over a long period of time. If she is psychiatrically ill, the likelihood of her developing further psychiatric symptoms after cosmetic surgery is high.

If there is no evidence of a psychiatric disorder, this should be explained to the surgeon, whose decision may be helped by some findings of the assessment (e.g. personality, social aspects/handicaps, attitude). Aspects such as the girl's expectations (e.g. she should not assume that cosmetic surgery of itself will solve her problems) and awareness of risks (e.g. scarring, altered sensation) should be discussed with him and balanced against the likely benefits (e.g. improved self-image and self-esteem). Even in the absence of preceding psychiatric symptoms, there is an increased likelihood of developing psychiatric morbidity after cosmetic surgery of this nature.

FURTHER READING

Committee on Safety of Medicines 1990 Cardiotoxic effects of pimozide. Current Problems 29

Harris D L 1989 The benefits and hazards of cosmetic surgery. British Journal of Hospital Medicine 41 (6): 540–545

Jenkins R, Shepherd M 1983 Mental illness and general practice. In: Bean P (ed) Mental illness: changes and trends. John Wiley & Sons, Chichester pp 379–409

Marks I, Mishan J 1988 Dysmorphophobic avoidance with disturbed bodily perception. A pilot study of exposure therapy. British Journal of Psychiatry 152: 674–678

Robin A A, Copas J B, Jack A B, Kaeser A C, Thomas P J 1988 Reshaping the psyche: the concurrent improvement in appearance and mental state after rhinoplasty. British Journal of Psychiatry 152: 539–543

A33

It is important to ascertain what the general practitioner means by 'confused'. Is the patient disorientated; has she got muddled thoughts, clouding of consciousness and other signs of an acute or subacute confusional state? What are the specific difficulties that are being encountered in terms of her behaviour? Is she believed to be a danger to herself, or is she putting other people at risk by her behaviour? Does she live alone, and if not with whom? Do any of her family members see her regularly?

The next issue to clarify is which of her family members do not want her to be seen by a psychiatrist, and why. Arrangements should be made to see the family in order to explore their motivations and fears, and to explore any family problems which may underlie their refusal. If the objection is to her being seen by a psychiatrist, they may accept a visit from other members of the clinical team who could carry out a home assessment.

If this fails, the general practitioner should be advised to carry out a detailed assessment of both her physical and mental state. Confusion may mean a general inability to think and act with one's customary clarity, may be used as a synonym for an acute organic brain syndrome (delirium), or may be used to mean both acute and chronic brain syndromes. Delirium may be precipitated by common physical conditions, such as pneumonia, cardiac failure, urinary infections, carcinomas or hypokalaemia, and by less common physical disorders. If the patient has a pre-existing cognitive impairment, relatively minor physical problems, such as constipation or dehydration, may precipitate delirium. Other causes of delirium include drug intoxication, withdrawal of drugs or alcohol, metabolic or endocrine disturbance, intracranial lesions, infections, head injury and vitamin deficiency.

If the cause of the acute organic brain syndrome is not easily elicited, the general practitioner should be advised to seek the help of the community geriatric physician. Drugs should generally be avoided in delirium, as impairment of consciousness may be increased. However, if the patient is overactive and disturbed, symptomatic relief can be provided with small doses of haloperidol, thioridazine or promazine. Benzodiazepines should be avoided because they may in-

crease the confusion. Chloral hydrate and dichloralphena-
zone (Welldorm) may be used if a hypnotic is needed.

The psychiatrist should be available for further consulta-
tion with the general practitioner or geriatric physician, with
the possibility of a joint assessment being carried out at a
later date.

FURTHER READING

Cutting J 1987 The phenomenology of acute organic psychosis: comparison
with acute schizophrenia. British Journal of Psychiatry 151: 324–332

Lipowski Z J 1984 Organic brain syndromes: new classification, concepts
and prospects. Canadian Journal of Psychiatry 29: 198–204

A34

The emergence of her symptoms following a stressful experience suggests the occurrence of a reactive disorder, where
her hand-washing could be one among other symptoms of a
depressive or anxiety reaction. The assessment will clarify
whether her obsessive symptoms are accompanied by other
symptoms of a depressive disorder, or are part of an obsessive-compulsive disorder.

Circumstances of onset must be explored: fear of con-
tamination, guilt that she may have been responsible for the
death of that patient, a grief reaction, etc. A functional analysis of her behaviour must be carried out, and the antecedents
and consequences of her hand-washing clearly established.
She should describe situations in which her hand-washing
occurs, e.g. at work, at home or at both; how frequent her behaviour is, e.g. everytime that she handles a patient, or
every 20 minutes; how incapacitating this is for her, e.g. problems at work, social handicaps; how long her hand-washing
takes, e.g. if it is a quick wash or if she spends several minutes
in a ritualised activity; if there are fluctuations, e.g. the frequency of her behaviour varies on different occasions; and
factors that make her problem worse or better.

Predisposing factors and features of an affective illness or
an obsessive-compulsive disorder in the past must be looked
for. The patient may have a history of obsessive symptoms
which were aggravated by the event in the ward. Obsessional
symptomatology may occur at the onset of organic brain dis-

order and in psychotic illnesses, and these conditions have to be considered.

If a depressive disorder is diagnosed, the nurse may be treated with psychotherapy (behavioural, cognitive, psychodynamic), and antidepressants may be helpful. She may need help to grieve the death of the patient.

If she is found to have an obsessive-compulsive disorder which was precipitated or aggravated by the experience, behavioural treatment, such as response prevention, would be indicated. Associated treatment with antidepressants may be beneficial. Serotonergic drugs, such as clomipramine and fluvoxamine, seem to be more effective in obsessive-compulsive disorder.

Behavioural psychotherapy can be given in the outpatient clinic through a self-exposure programme. After the nature of her problem is assessed in detail, a behavioural programme (exposure and response prevention) to produce improvement can be planned with her. If, for example, she washes her hands everytime that she touches a patient, her self-exposure 'homework' can be established as handling her patients as usual (exposure) and washing her hands only after she sees, say, five of them (response prevention). A colleague can help as a co-therapist. The tasks and their outcome (e.g. level of anxiety) should be recorded every-day in a diary. In the next session, she must bring the diary back for discussion and suggestions on how to proceed further (e.g. washing her hands only after she touches eight patients). She must be taught to anticipate setbacks and how to manage them. The process should continue until there is a sustained improvement.

FURTHER READING

Marks I M 1987 Behavioural psychotherapy in general psychiatry. Helping patients to help themselves. British Journal of Psychiatry 150: 593–597

Marks I M, Lelliott P, Basoglu M et al 1988 Clomipramine, self-exposure and therapist-aided exposure for obsessive-compulsive rituals. British Journal of Psychiatry 152: 522–534

Murphy D L, Zohar J, Benkelfat C, Pato M T, Pigott T A, Insel T R 1989 Obsessive-compulsive disorder as a 5-HT subsystem-related behavioural disorder. British Journal of Psychiatry 155 (suppl. 8): 15–24

A35

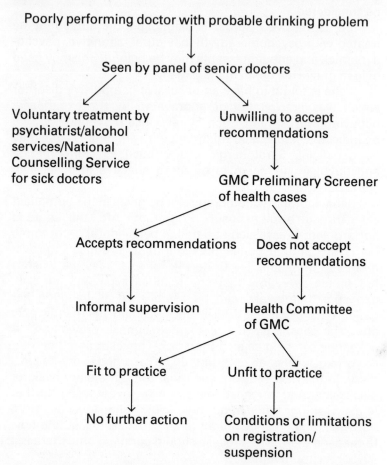

Poorly performing doctor with probable drinking problem

Seen by panel of senior doctors

Voluntary treatment by psychiatrist/alcohol services/National Counselling Service for sick doctors

Unwilling to accept recommendations

GMC Preliminary Screener of health cases

Accepts recommendations

Does not accept recommendations

Informal supervision

Health Committee of GMC

Fit to practice

Unfit to practice

No further action

Conditions or limitations on registration/ suspension

This doctor seems to have a drinking problem. It is important to establish first whether the doctor is or is not considered fit to work in terms of his performance and his responsibilities.

Within each Health District, there is a panel of senior doctors who act on behalf of the chief administrative doctor, i.e. chairman of the Medical Committee. Your colleague should approach these doctors, who may interview the doctor in question and submit a report to the administrative doctor on whether or not he is medically unfit to work.

If considered medically unfit to work, his willingness to acknowledge this and to accept treatment must be established.

Every effort should be made to persuade the doctor to seek some form of help voluntarily. If he accepts this suggestion, he may be referred to a psychiatrist or to the alcohol services. Alternatively, he may be referred to the National Counselling Service for sick doctors. This service has no statutory control. It operates a telephone hotline and has a network of advisors in all specialties, as well as counsellors. The advantage of this scheme is that it provides help from a source well outside the doctor's own district, thus assuring confidentiality. Referral to this scheme may be made by the colleague or the 'sick doctor' himself.

If the doctor is not willing to accept the judgment of his colleagues, his case might be referred to the General Medical Council. A referral of this kind would go to the Preliminary Screener of health cases, who would invite the doctor to be examined by doctors living near his home. If he complies with the recommendations regarding management and supervision, the matter is dealt with informally. If the doctor does not comply with the management recommended the case would then go before the Health Committee of the General Medical Council. This committee has the task of deciding whether the doctor's ability to practice is seriously impaired, and, if so, deciding on a course of action. This could include limiting his practice or suspending him.

FURTHER READING

Rawnsley K 1985 Helping the sick doctor: a new service. British Medical Journal 291: 922

Rawnsley K 1986 Sick doctors. Journal of the Royal Society of Medicine 79: 440–441

Kilpatrick R 1988 Helping the sick doctor : the work of the GMC's Health Committee. Journal of the Royal Society of Medicine 81: 436–437

A36

Female aged 16 years, overdose with 40 g of paracetamol, 8
hours ago.
Psychiatric assessment before discharge from casualty

$\downarrow$

SHOULD NOT BE DISCHARGED
- serious hepatic and other damage very likely
- serum levels do not indicate degree of damage
- physical signs often delayed

$\downarrow$

Appropriate medical treatment as an inpatient

$\downarrow$

Psychiatric assessment when appropriate:
- degree of suicidal intent and risk
- details of previous attempts
- psychosocial stressors and support systems
- other associated psychiatric problems

$\downarrow$

Treatment
- appropriate treatment and support
  (outpatient/inpatient care, community support,
  psychotherapy, etc.)

In a person who has taken 40 g of paracetamol, management
of physical complications takes precedence over the psy-
chatric assessment.

1. Paracetamol overdose
   - Hepatic damage likely if more than 8 g is taken as a
     single dose.
   - Plasma concentration of >200 μg/l, four hours after a
     dose implies that hepatic damage is very likely.
   - There may be no clinical or biochemical evidence of he-
     patic damage until 24–48 hours after ingestion.
   - Other complications include renal tubular necrosis,
     pancreatitis, hypoglycaemia, cardiac damage and
     hypersensitivity reactions.
   - Early clinical signs of toxicity are non-specific and in-

clude lethargy, pallor, nausea, vomiting and diaphoresis. Persistence of these signs beyond 24 hours, along with development of right subcostal pain and tenderness, usually indicates hepatocellular damage.
- An elevated serum transaminase could be the only early biochemical evidence of hepatic damage.
- Treatment of an overdose as large as 40 g should start with induction of emesis or gastric lavage if taken within four hours of presentation, and acetylcysteine/methionine therapy within 10–12 hours of ingestion.

One should ensure that appropriate treatment has been carried out. Observation and monitoring of the patient in hospital is *absolutely essential* in this case. Whatever the outcome of the psychiatric assessment, your recommendation should be that the patient is kept in hospital for medical reasons.

2. Psychiatric assessment may need to be delayed until physical complications are dealt with. The points listed below should be mentioned:

- Establish rapport with the patient and conduct the interview sensitively.
- The patient's explanation for the attempt and appraisal of its consequences at the time of the attempt should be obtained.
- Degree of suicidal intent at the time of the attempt (was the patient alone; were precautions taken against being discovered; was a suicide note written; was a will made; was she aware of the potential toxicity of paracetamol?).
- Details of previous attempts by the patient, the circumstances under which she threatened to kill herself, and how these were received by her family/boyfriend.
- Degree of social and psychological support available, current problems, social background, quality of relationship with parents and boyfriend, history of similar attempts by relatives or friends.
- Presence of any underlying physical or psychiatric problems, drug or alcohol abuse.
- Personality strengths and weaknesses, ability to cope with crises.
- Mental state examination.

The aims of assessment are to determine the risk of repetition, assess current problems that the patient needs help with, establish what further help is needed and who is best able to provide this. If she insists on discharging herself, she should be assessed for compulsory admission under Section 2 of the Mental Health Act (1983).

FURTHER READING

Friedman P A 1987 Poisoning and its management. In: Braunwald et al Harrison's principles of internal medicine. McGraw-Hill, London, pp 841–842

Hawton K, Catalan J 1987 Attempted suicide: a practical guide to its nature and management, 2nd ed. Oxford Medical Publications, Oxford

A37

45-year-old man with Hodgkin's disease; 'Difficult' and refusing treatment

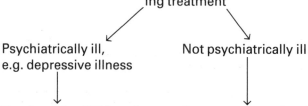

Psychiatrically ill, e.g. depressive illness

Not psychiatrically ill

Detain under MHA and treat

Cannot treat against his will

Hodgkin's disease is a physical condition which does not in itself warrant treatment against the patient's will. Nevertheless, the patient's refusal to accept treatment may be due to an independent psychiatric problem or to a complication of the primary physical condition. Psychiatric conditions which may be associated with Hodgkin's disease include depressive disorders, and agitation and confusional states.

Treatment depends on the detailed assessment of the patient and the problems.

The history should include past and current physical problems, medication, and previous psychiatric problems. Physical and mental examination, together with any special investigations available, will help elucidate the problems. Although it may not be very clear, an attempt should be made to establish whether any depressive disorder in this patient is a primary illness unrelated to Hodgkin's disease, is symptomatic of Hodgkin's disease or is a sequel to his Hodgkin's disease.

It is possible that there is no psychiatric problem and that the patient is angry, frustrated, fed-up or has just changed his mind about accepting further treatment. In the absence of any evidence of mental illness, it is not possible to enforce treatment.

If however, the disturbed behaviour is due to psychiatric disorder, either primary or secondary to a physical illness, it is possible to treat against the patient's will; as long as the behaviour is seen to put his health and/or his life at risk.

It is permissible, in an emergency, to treat the patient, without implementing the Mental Health Act. However, it is essential that the Mental Health Act Commission be informed and that the patient be formally detained under the Act as soon as possible in order to facilitate necessary and appropriate management.

FURTHER READING

Devlen J, Maguire P, Phillips P, Crowther D, Chambers H 1987 Psychological problems associated with diagnosis and treatment of lymphomas I: Retrospective study. British Medical Journal 295: 953–954

Devlen J, Maguire P, Phillips P, Crowther D 1987 Psychological problems associated with diagnosis and treatment of lymphomas II : prospective study. British Medical Journal 295: 955–957

A38

Details of the onset of the problem and changes in her behaviour will clarify whether or not the patient is presenting with a delusional belief of love, i.e. erotomania. Most cases of erotomania occur within the context of a primary psychiatric illness, most commonly schizophrenia or affective illness. Cases associated with drugs, senile dementia and organic delusional disorder have also been reported. She must, therefore, be carefully assessed for the presence of an underlying organic or psychiatric condition.

Pure erotomania, i.e. that which occurs in the absence of an associated psychiatric illness, seems to be uncommon. Classically, the patient, who is usually female, has a delusional belief that another person often of higher status, such as a superior at work, loves her intensely. She may, as in this case, become a nuisance or a threat towards the object of her love.

Treatment will be dictated by the nature of her disorder. Admission may be necessary for further assessment if the patient is socially and/or functionally disabled by her condition. It is essential to attend to the psychological distress that she may be experiencing. Antipsychotics may be helpful, and pimozide is said to be more effective than other antipsychotics. A complete physical evaluation must be carried out before pimozide is prescribed. Pure erotomania, however, is very resistant to medication or psychotherapy.

It is important to assess how she has responded to her superior's rebuff. She may feel resentful, and her love may have turned to anger and hatred. If she seems inclined to act on her feelings, the patient could be a danger to the wife, family or lover of her superior, who should be advised to take appropriate precautions. In this case, all resources available (e.g. medical adviser, general practitioner) should be used to monitor her behaviour and to determine how she might react. Her permission for the involvement of other agencies should be obtained.

FURTHER READING

Committee on safety of Medicines 1990 Cardiotoxic effects of pimozide. Current problems 29

Ellis P, Mellsop G 1985 De Clerambault's syndrome – a nosological entity? British Journal of Psychiatry 151: 400–402

Enoch M D, Trethowan W H 1979 Uncommon psychiatric syndromes, 2nd edn. Wright, Bristol

Signer S F, Swinson R P 1987 Two cases of erotomania (de Clerambault's syndrome) in bipolar affective disorder. British Journal of Psychiatry 151: 853–855

A 39

A. It is important to establish whether anybody has responsibility for the patient's ongoing care. This could be done by asking the patient, contacting the general practitioner, or contacting local day centres, day hospitals and social services. If he is not in receipt of ongoing care, or if this has broken down in some way, he has to have a detailed assessment of his physical and mental state as well as his social circumstances.

A detailed mental state examination is most important both for diagnostic purposes and to assess his functional capacities or lack of them.

The man's physical condition may warrant admission. If he is not admitted, the immediate issue that remains is still his physical wellbeing and his safety. Assessment of his social circumstances will have established whether or not he has accommodation. The reasons for his not wanting/being able to return to his residence may range from him having locked himself out, to having no gas or electricity, to not getting on with the neighbours. It may be possible to get him back home with the help of the local housing officer. If this is not possible, or if he has no accommodation, some form of emergency accommodation may have to be found. There should be a list of locally available night shelters or other hostels in the accident and emergency department or in the social work department. Additional advice should be sought from social work colleagues. The other immediate problems are those of food and money. He may have to be given some money from the emergency social fund to pay for food as well as for his overnight stay.

Having sorted out the issues of his immediate needs, some arrangements have to be made for his longer term care. He should be referred to a day hospital for a re-assessment of his long-term care needs. Here, he will be re-assessed in terms of his psychiatric and physical state, as well as his ability to live independently. The most appropriate type of accommodation should then be arranged in terms of his ability to cope on his own, interact with other people and manage a domestic environment. His ability to take care of his personal hygiene and his meals will also influence the type of living arrangements that are recommended, as will additional support that may be provided in terms of home help, and meals provided at the day centre or day hospital. Help with organising his finances may have to be provided. This may mean organising direct payment of bills as well as teaching him basic budgeting skills.

A range of daytime activities may be offered, depending on the patient's needs and level of functioning. This could be a fairly unstructured day centre or drop-in centre, or a highly structured work-like environment in a day hospital. Social support may be offered in the form of befrienders, social clubs, etc. Medication, if appropriate, may be given at the day centre, at home by the community psychiatric nurse or at the surgery by the general practitioner. It is important that somebody has responsibility for this patient. If not, he may get lost to the system again or get into trouble without anybody noticing.

B. The most likely cause of the man's frostbite is that he has been sleeping rough for some time and that he is suffering from the effects of the cold. Additionally, many of the major neuroleptics, such as chlorpromazine, produce hypothermia, so if he was taking medication this may have contributed to the development of frostbite.

FURTHER READING

Burns T P 1989 Community care and rehabilitation. Current Opinion in Psychiatry 2: 273–277

Shepherd G 1988 Practical aspects of management of negative symptoms. International Journal of Mental Health 16: 75–97

A40

A. Assessment:

1. Chromosomal abnormalities/risk factors:
– child: trisomy 21, translocation
– parents: age, carriers.

2. Family situation:
– child: age, handicap, condition/development
– parents: marital relationship, coping, psychiatric disorder
– other children: impact, difficulties
– support: social/financial, psychological.

B. Advice:

High risk – translocation: Low risk – regular trisomy: 1%

– 21/21: 100%
– others (e.g. 21/22): 5–20%

Amniocentesis + counselling

Factors which would make having another child inadvisable:

- poor marital relationship
- large family
- psychiatric disorder in parents or other family members, especially in the child with Down's syndrome
- seriously mentally handicapped child + difficulties in coping
- inadequate/poor social + financial + emotional support.

The first step is to make a genetic assessment. This involves the identification of the chromosomal abnormality and estimating the risk for the next child. If the Down's syndrome is due to a regular trisomy of chromosome 21, the risk of recurrence would be 1%. The risk is higher in case of trans-locations: 100% in the case of a translocation 21/21, and ranging from 5–20% in case of other translocations, such as 21/22. Father or mother can be the carriers of a translocation 21/21. Maternal age is another risk factor: Down's syndrome occurs in 1 in 660 of all births, but the proportion is 1 in 1050 for teenage mothers and 1 in 50 for mothers aged over 45. Paternal age may also be a significant risk factor for translocations.

It is important to assess how the couple have been coping with their child with Down's syndrome. Having a handicapped child involves problems and responsibilities which are often distressing, leading sometimes to reactions such as chronic grief which may be denied. For the parents, the birth is likely to have been a critical life experience. Amongst the parents of children with Down's syndrome, half of the couples show severe tension and high hostility between husband and wife, whereas the other half feel their marriage strengthened by the experience. If they have other children, the difficulties involved in having a handicapped brother or sister should be explored.

Information should be obtained on the level of impairment and the degree of disability of their child. It should be determined whether appropriate care is being provided for his/her needs and if provisions for his/her education have been arranged.

Ascertaining the level of care that the child requires at home is important, as this will have an impact on their ability to take care of a second child. It is also important to know whether the family have had access to the sources of support which are available, such as extra financial help, allocation of a social worker, schemes of help at home, respite care and self-help parent groups.

Following the genetic assessment, the conclusions can be discussed with the parents. They should be informed of the risks in terms that they can understand, and allowed to make their own decision. Advice will be given on the basis of what has been found. If the risk of Down's syndrome is low, conditions at home are favourable and they decide to have another child, an amniocentesis should be arranged in order to screen the next pregnancy. However, the couple will need counselling to help them to make a balanced decision if the amniocentesis shows that the second child also has Down's syndrome. On the other hand, the conclusions may be such that having another child at home, at least at this moment, would not be advisable, and postponement of the plan should be recommended.

FURTHER READING

Baraitser M 1986 Chromosomes and mental retardation (editorial). Psychological Medicine 16: 495–497

Gath A 1977 The impact of an abnormal child upon the parents. British Journal of Psychiatry 130: 405–410

Russel O 1985 Mental handicap. In: Paykel E S, Morgan H G (eds) Current Reviews in Psychiatry, Vol 1. Churchill Livingstone, Edinburgh

A41

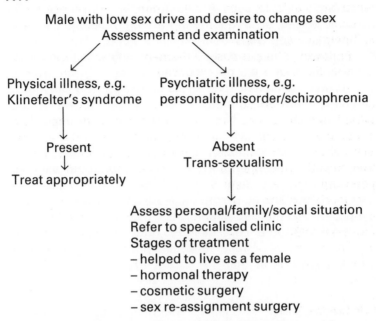

Male with low sex drive and desire to change sex
Assessment and examination

Physical illness, e.g.
Klinefelter's syndrome

Psychiatric illness, e.g.
personality disorder/schizophrenia

Present

Absent
Trans-sexualism

Treat appropriately

Assess personal/family/social situation
Refer to specialised clinic
Stages of treatment
– helped to live as a female
– hormonal therapy
– cosmetic surgery
– sex re-assignment surgery

This librarian appears to have an abnormality of gender identity. All sexual deviations can be manifestations of an underlying psychiatric disorder, and the first step, therefore, is to either rule out or establish the presence of a primary psychiatric of physical illness. There may be some difficulty in ascertaining whether or not this belief is delusional. The trans-sexual's belief is not delusional, as he/she *feels like* a member of the opposite sex rather than believing that he/she *is* a member of the opposite sex, and establishing this is crucial to the diagnosis. The opinion of a specialist should be sought if there are underlying endocrine, neurological or other physical problems.

The patient's 'low sex-drive' should be carefully explored. He could have a decreased libido or impaired sexual performance. One should find out his feelings about his external genitalia, and whether he is a practising homosexual or a heterosexual. His belief of mistaken gender identity could have developed within the context of other sexual problems, and treatment of the primary sexual problem may alter it. The consistency of the various manifestations of his belief, and the effect it has had on his social and sexual life should be evaluated. Substance abuse and problems with the law are more common than usual in this group, and these should be carefully looked for. Obtaining further information from other independent sources would facilitate appropriate management; however, in this case, if the patient wishes to maintain confidentiality, this will not be possible.

Further management depends on the primary diagnosis, and only the management of trans-sexualism will be discussed here. In establishing the diagnosis of trans-sexualism, it is useful to follow the DSM-III-R criteria, which state that there should be a persistent state of discomfort about one's assigned sex, and a persistent pre-occupation for at least two years with getting rid of one's primary and secondary sex characteristics and acquiring those of the opposite sex, after the person has reached puberty. The diagnosis should not be made if the disturbance is limited to brief periods of stress.

The treatment of trans-sexualism poses many clinical and ethical problems. If there is an underlying psychiatric disorder, then this should be treated first. The presence of a psychiatric disorder would usually contraindicate specific treatment for trans-sexualism. Treatment is best undertaken in specialised clinics and the individual should be referred to one. Before starting treatment, he should be advised about the effects a change of sex would have on his life. There may be complicated social and legal issues that he may need to consider, for example he may have fathered a child. He should be advised to obtain legal advice on such matters. Obtaining his consent to treatment is another important issue. Once it is established that there are no contraindications to treatment, and that the patient definitely wants to undergo treatment, the patient must be made fully aware of the details of treatment, and explicit written consent must be obtained.

There are three stages to the treatment of trans-sexualism in this person. In the first stage, he is helped to dress like, and develop behavioural traits and social skills of the female sex. Organizations exist that will give him valuable support and help him to come to terms with these changes. Supportive psychotherapy from a therapist skilled in this field can be invaluable. The patient should be given enough time to adjust to this role, as this real-life test could make him change his mind. In the next stage, he is given hormone therapy or cyproterone acetate, to help him develop female secondary sexual characteristics, provided there are no contraindications to their use. He should be aware of the fact that physical complications could arise and that the feminising effects of the drugs can be limited.

The third stage, sex-reassignment surgery (SRS), is an extremely controversial procedure, and will result in an irreversible change in his sexual characteristics. Before proceeding with surgery, it is important to be sure that surgery is absolutely indicated and that the patient has consented to it after being fully educated about the possible physical and psychological sequelae. If he adjusts well to a period of 'cross-dressing' and is fairly young, the outcome of SRS is more likely to be favourable. Any underlying psychiatric or medical problem could be a relative contraindication to SRS. Feminising surgery in this case will involve excision of the body of the penis, shortening the urethral tube and creating a simulated vaginal cavity, all of which are often associated with post-operative complications. Cosmetic surgery, such as breast augmentation, reduction of the thyroid cartilage and rhinoplasty, can help give him a feminine appearance. It is important that he is followed up carefully, as the outcome after SRS or, indeed, any of the above procedures may not be satisfactory.

FURTHER READING

Braude W M 1983 Management of sexual deviations. In: Berrios G E, Dowson J H (eds) Treatment and management in adult psychiatry. Balliere Tindall, London, ch. 23

Burns A, Farrell M, Christie-Brown J 1990 Clinical features of patients attending a gender-identity clinic. British Journal of Psychiatry 157: 265–268

Harry Benjamin International Gender Dysphoria Association 1985 Standards of care: the hormonal and surgical sex reassignment of gender dysphoric persons. Archives of Sexual Behaviour 14: 79–90

Lundstrom B, Pauly I, Walinder J 1984 Outcome of sex reassignment surgery. Acta Psychiatrica Scandinavica 70: 289–294

Mate-Kole C, Freschi M, Robin A 1990 A controlled study of psychological and social change after surgical gender reassignment in selected male transsexuals. British Journal of Psychiatry 157: 261–264

Randell J 1971 Indications for sex-reassignment surgery. Archives of Sexual Behaviour, 1 (2): 153–161

A42

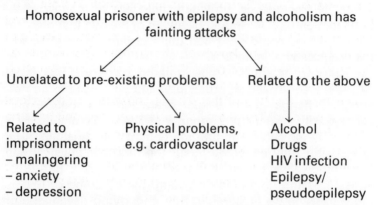

Homosexual prisoner with epilepsy and alcoholism has fainting attacks

Unrelated to pre-existing problems

Related to the above

Related to imprisonment
– malingering
– anxiety
– depression

Physical problems, e.g. cardiovascular

Alcohol
Drugs
HIV infection
Epilepsy/ pseudoepilepsy

The fainting attacks could be unrelated to the epilepsy or alcoholism, but could be due to physical problems such as cardiovascular disorders, or psychiatric problems such as anxiety or depression. The other possibilities to be considered are that the patient may be malingering or may have Ganser's syndrome. However, it is more likely that the attacks are related to the consequences of alcohol abuse, i.e. malnutrition or hepatic failure or other conditions, such as epilepsy or HIV infection.

Treatment is dependent on the underlying cause and has to be preceded by a careful assessment in order to establish a diagnosis.

The first step is to ascertain the details of the fainting attacks: when they developed; whether they occur at particular times, e.g. standing abruptly; how long they last for; whether they are preceded by particular events, e.g. being asked to do something; whether they are associated with any other features, e.g. frothing at the mouth; whether the patient ever injures himself during these attacks, etc. A history should also be taken from any of the prison staff who have witnessed these attacks. A generalised seizure will be characterised by sudden onset, tonic then clonic convulsions, followed by profound unconsciousness for several minutes at least. The patient may have bitten his tongue or been incontinent of urine during the attacks. Examination during the attacks may have revealed absent corneal reflexes and extensor plantar responses. Post-ictal states may include disorientation, severe headache and, occasionally, psychotic phenomena. Pseudoseizures tend to occur only in front of an audience, but the patient may appear to be unconscious and may move his arms and legs in the manner characteristic of generalised epilepsy. However, the corneal and plantar reflexes would have been normal. Akinetic seizures, characterised by the sudden and profound loss of muscular tone, would have resulted in the patient collapsing unconscious without warning. These only last a few seconds and have no after effects except the high risk of injury. As these drop attacks are thought to represent brief attentuated forms of seizure discharges in patients with grand mal epilepsy, looking for these would be particularly important in this patient.

Family history should be explored for evidence of cardiac conditions or diabetes, as his syncope may be due to arrhythmias or hypoglycaemia.

All details of his alcohol abuse, his epilepsy and any treatment that he received for these conditions should be ascertained, as this may be underlying his present complaint. This would also be important for the new treatment plan. It would be important, too, to establish whether the patient is at risk of developing HIV infection, or whether he believes that he has HIV infection. A detailed physical examination should be carried out. Examination of his mental state may reveal signs of anxiety or depression.

Further investigations would include getting details of his previous history from his general practitioner and hospital records, if possible. Haematological and biochemical examination may reveal evidence of liver dysfunction, anaemia, infections, hypoglycaemia and drug abuse. Skull X-ray may demonstrate head injury, EEG may demonstrate continuing seizures and an ECG may reveal cardiac dysfunction. HIV testing may only be carried out with the patient's consent, after counselling.

Most of these investigations may be done in prison. However, some specialised investigations, such as the EEG, may require that he be transferred to hospital. Treatment will depend on the cause of the attacks and will be the responsibility of the prison medical officer. Advice should be given to the prison medical officer and the prison hospital staff (if appropriate) on both the assessment and the treatment.

If treatment has to be carried out in a hospital, then the issue of his transfer to hospital arises. For a detailed discussion of transfer of prisoners to hospital, see Q24.

FURTHER READING

Fenton G W 1983 Epilepsy. In: Lader M H (ed) Handbook of psychiatry, 2nd edn. Cambridge University Press, Cambridge

Laidlaw J, Richens A, Oxley J (eds) 1988 A textbook of epilepsy. Churchill Livingstone, Edinburgh

A43

19-year-old girl with altered body image, bingeing and induced vomiting after leaving home and taking up employment.

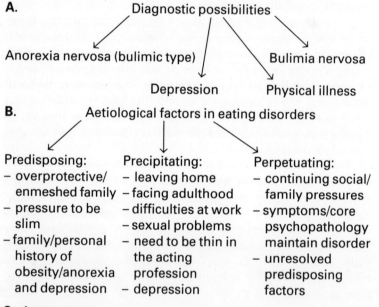

A.   Diagnostic possibilities

Anorexia nervosa (bulimic type)   Bulimia nervosa

Depression   Physical illness

B.   Aetiological factors in eating disorders

Predisposing:	Precipitating:	Perpetuating:
– overprotective/ enmeshed family	– leaving home	– continuing social/ family pressures
– pressure to be slim	– facing adulthood	– symptoms/core psychopathology maintain disorder
– family/personal history of obesity/anorexia and depression	– difficulties at work	– unresolved predisposing factors
	– sexual problems	
	– need to be thin in the acting profession	
	– depression	

C. Assessment

- general psychopathology: depression, personality, impaired social/sexual functioning, guilt, anger, denial and neurotic traits
- core psychopathology: altered body image, behaviour to control body weight

- family environment/pathology, social environment
- body weight, menstrual pattern, associated physical problems.

D. Treatment (Bulimia nervosa):

- outpatient usually
- inpatient if physically ill, suicidal
- cognitive-behavioural therapy
- individual/group psychotherapy
- antidepressants if depressed/medical treatment for physical problems
- consider change in occupation if child at risk.

The symptoms indicate either anorexia nervosa of the bulimic type, or bulimia nervosa. Weight loss as a result of extreme dieting and other behaviour to control weight, amenorrhea and an altered body image, in addition to bulimic episodes, would suggest anorexia nervosa of the bulimic type. As anorexia nervosa has been discussed elsewhere, this question will deal only with bulimia nervosa (BN). Symptoms that would suggest BN include an altered body image, overvalued ideas about her shape and weight, and loss of control over eating with bouts of excessive eating, i.e. bulimia. In addition to vomiting after meals, the patient may be using other methods to control her weight, such as severe dieting, use of laxatives and diuretics and exercising. She may or may not have weight loss or menstrual irregularity. Most women with BN present in their late teens or early twenties. The keeping of a 'diary' of food consumption and vomiting would help in diagnosis and treatment. It is important to look for underlying depression. Depending on the severity of her symptoms, there may be physical complications. These include weakness, gastro-oesophageal reflux, salivary gland enlargement, erosion of dental enamel due to repeated vomiting, callouses on the dorsal surface of the hand caused by using the fingers to induce vomiting, and electrolyte and metabolic abnormalities due to the use of laxatives and diuretics and repeated vomiting.

Aetiological factors and assessment are covered in the flow diagram. There is usually no reluctance to seek help, but if there is, the first step is to gain the patient's trust and persuade her to accept treatment. Treatment is usually carried out on an outpatient basis. In this case, it may be appropriate that she return home for the period of treatment. For example, she may be finding it very difficult to be away from home, and this could adversely affect the outcome of her treatment; or family involvement could prove essential. The absence of family problems, and a mild form of BN, may make outpatient treatment feasible, in the city. Inpatient treatment is only indicated if there are significant physical problems that need medical treatment, if the patient is very depressed and/or suicidal and if she does not respond to outpatient treatment. If her illness is interfering with her capacity to take care of her employers' child, she should be advised to give up working as an au pair for the time being.

The most widely used treatment methods include a combination of behavioural, cognitive and psychodynamic psychotherapy. The aims of treatment would be to modify the patient's abnormal body image and eating habits, and to improve her self-esteem. Cognitive-behavioural therapy lasts for about five months, and involves the use of various cognitive techniques to modify psychopathology and behaviour. The supervised consumption of food that is eaten during a bulimic episode (usually carbohydrate-rich), followed by the prevention of further eating or vomiting is a form of 'exposure with response prevention', and is successful in some patients. Antidepressants would be indicated only if she has significant underlying depression; they are of no use in the absence of depression. The continuing presence of any predisposing factors would increase the risk of reappearance of her symptoms after successful treatment. It is important, therefore, to address these factors and to ensure adequate follow-up.

FURTHER READING

Beaumont P J V 1988 Recent advances concerning eating disorders. Current Opinion In Psychiatry 1: 155–164

Fairburn C G, Cooper Z, Cooper P J 1986 The clinical features and maintenance of bulimia nervosa. In: Brownell K D, Foreyt J P (eds) Handbook of eating disorders; physiology, psychology, and treatment of obesity, anorexia and bulimia. Basic Books, New York

Garner D M, Garfinkel P E (eds) 1985 Handbook of psychotherapy for anorexia nervosa and bulimia. Guildford Press, New York

Striegel-Moore R H, Silberstein L R, Rodin J 1986 Towards an understanding of risk factors for bulimia. American Psychologist 41: 246

See also Q5

A44

This is a middle-aged woman whose complaint of abdominal pain does not appear to be associated with an organic illness. A history of sudden onset of her pain, the pain becoming worse with time and the symptom being inconsistent with the anatomical distribution of the sensory nervous system is suggestive of psychogenic pain (somatoform pain disorder). Other conditions, such as irritable bowel syndrome, should be considered.

The onset and course of the woman's pain must be explored. For example, it may have started after her children left home, following a physical illness or during menopause. The reason for her being referred now, after years with the symptom, should be explored, e.g. recent life event, worsening of the pain, other symptoms. Secondary gain may be identified, e.g. attention from relatives, a particular role within her family. The consequences of the pain should be established. Symptoms of depression, if present, may have started before or after the onset of the pain. It is important to know how disabling the pain is for her, e.g. is it preventing her from having a normal life?

Most patients with chronic somatic problems are convinced that they have a physical condition, and are often unwilling to accept a psychological explanation. The results of her physical investigations should be fully discussed with her. Great care should be taken to ensure that there are no implications that her symptoms are imaginary. It should be emphasised that, whatever the underlying cause of her pain, psychological treatment can help to alleviate her distress. Sympathetic concern towards the patient, attending closely to what she says and avoiding jargon, will be essential to achieve her compliance with the treatment.

Treatment should be aimed towards rehabilitation rather than cure of the pain, and will include:

- Individual and family interviews, in which precipitating or sustaining factors (marital or family discord, personality problems) should be identified.
- Investigations for underlying depression, anxiety or an undetected organic illness.
- Psychotherapy (e.g. family therapy, cognitive-behavioural methods) and/or pharmacological treatment (e.g. antidepressants).
- Regular appointments for reassurance and supportive psychotherapy, preferably with the same psychiatrist.
- Putting the patient in contact with self-help groups of people suffering chronic pain for group support, advice and counselling, such as SHIP (Self Help In Pain).
- If the pain is severe and relatively refractory to outpatient psychiatric treatment, she should be referred to a specialised pain relief clinic. Inpatient treatment may be indicated. These clinics use a multidisciplinary approach (anaesthetists, psychologists, psychiatrists, physiotherapists) and some of them adopt behavioural methods of management.

FURTHER READING

Creed F H 1990 Functional abdominal pain. In: Bass C (ed) Somatization: physical symptoms and psychological illness. Blackwell, London pp 141–170

Elton D, Stanley G, Burrows G 1983 Psychological control of pain. Grune and Stratton, London

Mayou R A 1988 Psychiatric treatment of somatic symptoms. Current Opinion in Psychiatry 1: 150–154

A45

A.   Acute organic reaction in a man, three days after admission with poor memory, disturbed behaviour, convulsions, nystagmus and opthalmoplegia

'Delirium'

Differential diagnosis

- Wernicke's encephalopathy
- head injury
- drug-induced (steroids/salicylates)
- epilepsy
- hepatic encephalopathy
- alcohol or drug withdrawal
- hypoglycaemia
- uraemia/electrolyte imbalance
- cardiovascular/ cerebrovascular problems
- meningitis/other infections

B.   Treatment of delirium with possible Wernicke's encephalopathy

Nursing
- bed rest in well-lit, uncluttered room
- monitor pulse/BP/ temperature
- intake/output chart
- adequate hydration (oral/intravenous)

Specific therapeutic measures
- fluid replacement
- adequate sedation
- high potency vitamins
- anticonvulsants
- treat underlying complications

The onset of symptoms a few days after admission, the history of an accident or fall, the patient's disturbed state and the occurrence of an epileptic fit suggest delirium tremens after abrupt withdrawal from alcohol. The presence of nystagmus and opthalmoplegia in addition suggest Wernicke's encephalopathy.

A complete account of the patient's presentation, treatment so far and the development of his current disturbed state should be obtained. A thorough neurological, cognitive and mental state examination should be carried out, keeping the various causes of an acute organic state in mind. The presence of ataxia, ophthalmoplegia, nystagmus, nausea and impaired memory would suggest Wernicke-Korsakoff syndrome. The red cell transketolase level should be investigated (before any parenteral vitamins are used) to look for thiamine deficiency. He could also have any of the other conditions listed in the flow diagram, perhaps in addition to the Wernicke-Korsakoff syndrome, and should be carefully investigated for these. An undetected head injury is particularly likely as he had a fall, and he should have a CT scan of his head. Other investigations that should be carried out are an electrolyte screen, a total and differential white blood cell count, haemoglobin, ESR, blood picture, platelet count, blood culture and, if indicated, a cerebrospinal fluid analysis.

Treatment of delirium tremens is outlined in the flow diagram. Adequate sedation is essential and the drug of choice is chlordiazepoxide, which can be given in doses up to 400 mg or more per day. Initial doses can be given intramuscularly, and if rapid sedation is necessary, intravenous diazepam may be used. High potency B vitamins (e.g. 'parenterovite') should be used for Wernicke's encephalopathy. If these are not available, then thiamine should be administered, 50 mg intravenously and 50 mg intramuscularly. The latter should be repeated daily until the patient resumes a normal diet, after which oral B vitamin supplements can be given. Intravenous glucose preparations given to alcoholic patients can severely deplete their reserve of B vitamins, and either precipitate Wernicke's disease or cause a rapid worsening of the condition. Anticonvulsants should be used in the short term to prevent any further seizures. The prevention and aggressive treatment of complications, such as dehydration, cardiovascular collapse, respiratory depression and infections, is essential. These complications, which are frequently present, are responsible for the high mortality rate in delirium tremens. After recovery from the acute episode, the patient should be assessed for any residual neurological and cognitive deficits, and appropriate rehabilitation offered. The problem of alcohol abuse should be dealt with, and his family should be closely involved at all stages of treatment and rehabilitation.

FURTHER READING

Castaneda R, Cusham P 1989 Alcohol withdrawal: a review of clinical management. Journal of Clinical Psychiatry 50: 278–284

Chick J 1989 Delirium tremens (Editorial) British Medical Journal 298: 3

Lipowski Z J 1984 Organic brain syndromes: new classification, concepts and prospects. Canadian Journal of Psychiatry 29: 198–204

Victor M, Adams R D, Collins G H 1971 The Wernicke Korsakoff Syndrome. Blackwell Scientific, Oxford

A46

The patient's chest pain and headaches could be associated with an undetected physical pathology. Therefore, it is essential to ascertain what investigations have been carried out and by whom (e.g. general practitioner, specialist). These symptoms may be part of an anxiety disorder, of a depressive illness, of an anxiety state with depressive phenomena or of a grief reaction with symptoms of depression and anxiety.

The onset and course of the patient's symptoms should be carefully investigated. It may be found, for example, that her mother's existence provided the main focus in her life so that now she feels without purpose and depressed (hence extra work at the school). On the other hand, her mother's death may have aggravated previously present symptoms of anxiety. Other factors (e.g. relationships, problems at work) may also be involved. Therefore, details of her personality and life style before her mother's death should be obtained.

The patient should be encouraged to talk about her mother, how she feels now that her mother is dead and the changes that she has experienced since her death. The details surrounding her death should be recalled. What were the conspicuous features of the relationship and interactions between the patient and her mother, especially in the months before her death? What were the circumstances of her death – was it unexpected or following a chronic illness; at home or in hospital? Was she present or not at the time? The details of her bereavement should be ascertained. Did she experience the pain of grief at all, or was the pain overwhelming? How long after her mother's death did she start grieving? Could she accept the reality of the loss, or does she still feel as if her mother is alive or may return? Has she adjusted to the environment in which her mother is missing?

Details of the patient's life with her mother should be explored. Their relationship could have been an ambivalent or a dependent one. A grief reaction may have occurred in the past at the death of her father. A depressive disorder may have passed undetected. She should be asked about her social network. It is important to know if she can count on support (e.g. from friends or relatives) or feels isolated. If an abnormal grief reaction is present, features such as self-blame and feelings of anger and guilt may be elicited. Hallucinations or illusions of her dead mother may occur.

If a physical illness is diagnosed, appropriate treatment should be arranged. In case the patient is found to have a depressive disorder, treatment could include psychotherapy and antidepressants. If she has an anxiety disorder, anxiety management training or behavioural/cognitive therapy could be helpful. However, if the disorder is most appropriately construed as an abnormal grief reaction; grief therapy is indicated. In grief therapy, a therapeutic contract must be set up with her. Memories of her mother should be revived (e.g. by talking about her mother, recalling situations), and those aspects of her grief process which have not been completed must be assessed (e.g. if her grief was absent, or if she was unable to reinvest her emotional energy in another relationship). She should be encouraged to express the affect which is associated with her memories (e.g. guilt, anger, tenderness, ambivalence). Linking objects (e.g. photographs, gifts) can be used to explore and to defuse her feelings. At the appropriate stage, she must be helped to acknowledge the finality of the loss (e.g. her mother will not return) and to face the end of her grieving (e.g. fears, resuming life, plans). The therapy will be completed with a final goodbye (e.g. a visit to her mother's grave).

FURTHER READING

Bass C 1990 Assessment and management of patients with functional somatic complaints. In: Bass C (ed) Somatization: physical symptoms and psychological illness. Blackwell, London

Clayton P J, Herjanic M, Murphy G E, Woodruff R 1974 Mourning and
  depression: their similarities and differences. Journal of the Canadian
  Psychiatric Association 19: 309–312

Parkes C M 1972 Bereavement: studies of grief in adult life. Tavistock,
  London

Worden J W 1983 Grief counselling and grief therapy. Tavistock, London

A47

This seems to be a problem of inappropriate sexual behaviour in an adolescent boy with mental retardation. The first step is to ascertain the nature and degree of mental retardation. This should be done by acquiring any information already available on this patient. All records of previous assessments and management should be obtained from his previous doctors, psychologists and school. The next task is to take a detailed history of the problem. Any antecedents to the behaviour should be ascertained, e.g. recent sex education in school. The details of the behaviour itself should be established, such as whether he had an erection or whether he masturbated. The response of the people around to his behaviour should be obtained, both the immediate response in the shop and that of his parents and family at home. His behaviour since then should also be determined. A clear picture should be obtained of the family situation, including physical and psychiatric disorder in the parents, and parental discord. His level of educational attainment and any previous behavioural or psychiatric difficulties should be ascertained. The recent move may be an important source of stress for him as well as for other members of his family.

Physical examination should reveal signs of puberty, and those of any organic disorders. Examination of his mental state may reveal evidence of anxiety, depression or psychosis, as well as cognitive deterioration. His current level of functioning must be compared with the previous reports obtained, in order to establish any deterioration of functioning.

Management will be aimed at any underlying problems, as well as the inappropriate sexual behaviour. Any major psychiatric problem should be treated, taking into account the increased side-effects with psychotropic drugs in mental impairment. If his behaviour is related to stress, such as change in school, the management should be aimed at reducing the stress, for example by working with the teachers in the school. Management of the inappropriate sexual behaviour should include an educational and behavioural approach. This should be done through the school. Inappropriate behaviour should not be reinforced, and if necessary he should have 'time out' until the behaviour subsides. Appropriate behaviour should be rewarded. There should be close collaboration between the school and the parents in order that any programme may be carried out in a coordinated manner. The parents should be reassured about his behaviour. Additional support should be provided for the family if necessary. This may take the form of behavioural training, parent group counselling or family therapy.

FURTHER READING

Hollins S C 1989 The family and the mentally handicapped person. Current Opinion in Psychiatry 2: 623–628

A48

From the description, this patient may have grand mal seizures, pseudoseizures or both. Typically, grand mal seizures start with sudden loss of consciousness followed by tonic-clonic convulsions. The patients frequently fall and injure themselves during these attacks and may also be incontinent of urine. After the attack, the patient may have a headache, be confused or behaviourally disturbed. Pseudoseizures, on the other hand, tend to occur in front of an audience and the patients usually do not injure themselves.

A history of these episodes of falling with convulsions should be obtained independently from a relative or a friend. Circumstances in which the seizures occur should be established. All seizures can occur in situations of increased stress. Pseudoseizures are said to occur more often in situations where the patient seeks to attract attention. It is important to establish whether there is a family history of epilepsy and, if there is, details should be elicited. A history of birth trauma or any other brain injury might be predisposing factors. The assessment of the patient's psychosocial and family situation should include aspects such as the family dynamics (e.g. family disharmony, how the family respond to her attacks), how the convulsions have affected her life (e.g. secondary gain and/or disabilities), sexual maladjustment, her difficulties at work and the presence of stressful life events. Physical examination may reveal evidence of injury sustained during seizures. A complete mental state examination should be carried out to establish the presence of any intercurrent psychiatric problems, which could range from anxiety to psychosis.

Previous investigations should be reviewed and, if necessary, further investigations carried out. In epilepsy, an interseizure EEG would probably show slow spikes, sharp waves and complexes, but abnormalities may also occur in other conditions, such as personality disorder and schizophrenia. If possible, an ictal and a post-ictal EEG should be obtained. Provocative techniques (e.g. overbreathing, photic stimulation, induced sleep and sleep deprivation) can be used. If necessary, continuous ambulatory EEG monitoring over 24 hours can be performed. Other techniques include simultaneous EEG and telemetry. Post-seizure prolactin levels should be measured as they would not be high in pseudoseizures, whereas they are always raised following true seizures.

Treatment will depend on the conclusion of the assessment. If the occurrence of tonic-clonic seizures is confirmed, treatment would include:

1. Medication: carbamazepine and/or phenytoin are the treatment of choice. Sodium valproate can also be used. Drugs should be started at a low dose and be gradually increased. If necessary, both drugs can be used in combination, although polypharmacy should be avoided. Monitoring of medication includes:

- clinical response
- side-effects (phenytoin – nystagmus, ataxia, mental changes, coarse facies, acne, hirsutism, gingival hyperplasia; carbamazepine – dizziness, drowsiness, gastro-intestinal disturbances, double vision, erythematous rash, leucopenia)
- drug levels (carbamazepine 4–12 mg/l, phenytoin 10–20 mg/l).

2. Psychological and social interventions: regular follow-up as an outpatient, counselling, support and reassurance are essential. Formal psychotherapy may provoke anxiety and aggravate the seizures. If there are family problems, a period

away from home may improve the situation. Counselling of relatives and employers is important. Advice should be given on matters such as sporting activities, alcohol intake and driving. The patient should be put in contact with self-help groups or agencies, such as the British Epilepsy Association.

If the patient is found to have non-epileptic seizures, any contributing or maintaining factors should be addressed. The patient might be helped to learn how to control her attacks. Anxiety-relieving techniques and psychotherapy (e.g. behavioural, group or family therapy) could be beneficial. A short admission should be considered to remove the patient from external environmental stressors, and for detailed assessment of psychosocial problems associated with the pseudoseizures.

FURTHER READING

Porter R J 1984 Epilepsy: 100 elementary principles. In Walton J N (ed) Major problems in neurology, Vol. 12. W B Saunders, London

Hermann B P, Whitman S, Wyler A R, Anton M T, Vanderzwagg R 1990 Psychological predictors of psychopathology in epilepsy. British Journal of Psychiatry 156: 98–105

A49

Fear of heart attack, chest pain and breathlessness in a 31-year-old bus driver

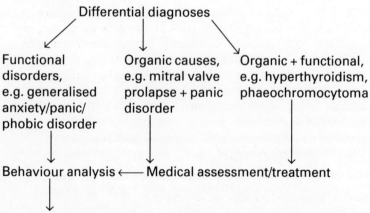

Differential diagnoses

Functional disorders, e.g. generalised anxiety/panic/phobic disorder

Organic causes, e.g. mitral valve prolapse + panic disorder

Organic + functional, e.g. hyperthyroidism, phaeochromocytoma

Behaviour analysis ←—— Medical assessment/treatment

Psychological treatment, e.g. behavioural/cognitive therapy, anxiety management

These symptoms may be caused by a physical illness, a psychological problem or both. The patient should be investigated for conditions such as hyperthyroidism, hypoglycaemia, phaeochromocytoma and mitral valve prolapse. Use of drugs (e.g. amphetamines) or excessive use of caffeine must be considered.

A history in which anxiety symptoms – somatic and psychological – are the predominant feature, especially if they are found to be associated with certain situations, would suggest an anxiety disorder. A detailed account of the onset, frequency, duration and fluctuation of the symptoms must be obtained. A history of panic attacks – hyperventilation, chest pain and other symptoms, such as palpitations, sweating, flushes and fear of dying – occurring in association with exposure to situations which provoke fear (e.g. crossing Waterloo bridge) would suggest panic disorder/agoraphobia. A history of continuous apprehension, muscle tension, restlessness, palpitations and irritability for several months would suggest a generalised anxiety disorder. These symptoms may also be a manifestation of an underlying depressive disorder.

Further management will be determined by the nature of the problem. If an underlying organic condition is detected, it should be treated. Admission may be indicated for further assessment or because the patient is severely disabled by his symptoms. The treatment of choice for anxiety, panic and phobic disorders is behavioural management. This may include cognitive therapy, exposure, or a combination of exposure with cognitive restructuring, especially if there is avoidance behaviour. In the absence of any avoidance, cognitive therapy, relaxation and anxiety management training would be indicated. Antidepressants, particularly imipramine and phenelzine, have been shown to be useful in generalised anxiety and panic disorders.

FURTHER READING

Basoglu M, Marks I 1989 Anxiety, panic and phobic disorders. Current Opinion in Psychiatry 2: 235–239

Bass C, Chambers J B, Kiff P, Cooper D, Gardner W P 1988 Panic anxiety and hyperventilation in patients with chest pain: a controlled study. Quarterly Journal of Medicine, 69: 949–959

Margrar J, Enlers A, Roth W I 1988 Mitral valve prolapse and panic disorder: a review of their relationship. Psychosomatic Medicine 50(2): 93–113

Marks I 1986 Behavioural psychotherapy: Maudsley pocket book of clinical management. Wright, Bristol

Marks I, O'Sullivan G 1988 Drugs and psychological treatments for agoraphobia, panic and obsessive-compulsive disorders: a review. British Journal of Psychiatry 151: 535–542

Pasnau R O 1984 Diagnosis and treatment of anxiety disorders. American Psychiatric Press, Washington D.C.

A50

From the description of this case, this woman appears to have hypomania. Despite the clear history of manic-depressive illness, possibilities such as hypomania secondary to physical illness or drug-induced psychosis should be considered. The immediate problem is to assess the severity of her hypomania and to see whether admission is needed, formally or informally. Compulsory admission would be indicated if she is putting herself at risk, or if the history suggests that she will shortly develop a much more serious manic illness.

Precipitating factors for the relapse of the woman's illness could include:

- Drugs: a careful drug history should be taken – dosage of each, compliance with drug taking. Relapse may have been precipitated by the woman discontinuing her drugs. She may have been prescribed other drugs, such as steroids or antiparkinsonian drugs, in addition to antipsychotic or mood stabilising drugs.
- Physical problems: a thorough physical examination should be done, but this may prove difficult in a patient who is hypomanic and may have to be postponed until she is more settled.
- Life events: the woman's symptoms may have been precipitated by a recent life event, such as death of a relative or a friend. There may be friction between the patient and the staff or other residents.

If treatment as an outpatient is indicated, this should include:

- Medication: getting manic patients to take medication is a risky business and unlikely to be successful. It will be necessary, therefore, to arrange adequate supervision of her medication by a community psychiatric nurse, a district nurse or other carers, such as a relative. Treatment could include lithium and/or oral or depot neuroleptics, depending on what is the most suitable regime for her. The risks involved in using these drugs in the elderly must be carefully considered.

- Advice to the staff: explaining about the illness, strategies of coping and avoiding distress would be helpful. Regular follow-up in the outpatient clinic or at home should be arranged.
- Practical help: if necessary, domestic, social and financial support should be provided with the assistance of a social worker.

FURTHER READING

Janiceck P G, O'Connor E 1990 Major affective disorders: issues involving recovery and recurrence. Current Opinion in Psychiatry 3: 48–53

Silverstone T, Romans-Clarkson S 1989 Bipolar affective disorders: causes and prevention of relapse. British Journal of Psychiatry 154: 321–335

A51

Orofacial dyskinesia in a woman with schizophrenia on maintenance neuroleptics

↓

Assessment
- neurological/physical examination
- mental state examination
- drugs taken since start of neuroleptic medication
- risk factors for tardive dyskinesia
- vulnerability to relapse after starting new job

↙   ↘

Tardive dyskinesia
- reduce neuroleptics to minimum effective dose
- avoid anticholinergics
- avoid drug holidays
- cholinergic agonists *may* help

Other movement disorders, e.g. familial chorea

↓

Treat accordingly

This woman, who is currently well, on depot medication, appears to be developing early signs of tardive dyskinesia (TD).

Having just started a job, she may also be vulnerable to a relapse of her underlying illness. One has to first ascertain whether she has TD and then decide on the best way to prevent a worsening of her symptoms.

The onset, nature and duration of any uncontrollable movements should be noted, including akathisia, which is often present along with TD. Family history of movement disorders should be looked for. Characteristic signs of TD are buccolingual masticatory movements, orofacial and limb dyskinesia and choreoathetoid movements. The exact dosage and frequency of her current depot and oral medication should be determine, including any she may be taking on an 'as required' basis.

If it seems from the assessment that the woman may be developing TD, she should be told that the facial twitch may be related to her medication in such a way as not to cause her undue alarm. Information on TD should be given, stressing the fact that often it is not progressive and that spontaneous remission may occur. The twitch could also be unrelated to her medication (e.g. idiopathic orofacial dyskinesia). Her current medication should be rationalised (minimum required dosage of neuroleptics, avoid using anticholinergics and multiple drugs), and the rationale underlying this explained to her. All anticholinergic and neuroleptic medication should be gradually reduced to the minimum effective dosage, and the woman should be warned about the temporary worsening in her twitch that could be brought about by this. Whatever reduction is clinically indicated at this stage should be made, and an early appointment given. If it is felt that she may have another movement disorder, she should be referred to a neurologist for a second opinion.

Between her appointments, a careful analysis should be made of her notes. All her episodes and the medication she has had over the years should be documented, and her response to any changes in medication, and vulnerability to relapse noted. The presence of 'negative' symptoms should be noted as they increase the risk of TD developing.

Long-term treatment consists of; prescribing the minimum effective dose of the neuroleptic and continuing the prescription only if there is clear benefit; using anticholinergics only if absolutely essential; and avoiding 'drug' holidays. (Recent research evidence shows that, contrary to earlier belief, drug holidays may in fact increase a patient's susceptibility to TD, as they would increase the total amount of neuroleptics that a patient would receive if he/she relapses as a result). For similar reasons, the risk of relapse should be carefully assessed when reducing neuroleptic dosage, as a relapse is not only undesirable but could also lead to the patient getting higher doses of the neuroleptic in future. There is no clear evidence linking specific drugs with TD, but the high-potency neuroleptics and fluphenazine decanoate appear to be associated more frequently than others. Specific D2 blockers (sulpiride) are said to lower the risk of TD developing, but there is little evidence to support this. Cholinergic agonist treatment (choline, deanol, lecithin) may reduce the severity of the TD.

FURTHER READING

Barnes T R E 1988 Tardive dyskinesia: risk factors, pathophysiology and treatment. In: Granville-Grossman K (ed) Recent advances in clinical psychiatry, Vol 6. Churchill Livingstone, Edinburgh, pp 185–207

Glazer W M, Bowers M B Jr, Charney D S, Heninger G R 1989 The effect of neuroleptic discontinuation on psychopathology, involuntary movements, and biochemical measures in patients with persistent tardive dyskinesia. Biological Psychiatry 26(3): 224–233

Yassa R 1989 Functional impairment in tardive dyskinesia; medical and psychosocial dimensions. Acta Psychiatrica Scandinavica 89(1): 64–67

A52

A.   Teenage girl, acutely psychotic after a RTA, was raped a year ago

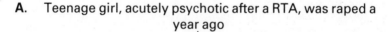

Differential diagnosis

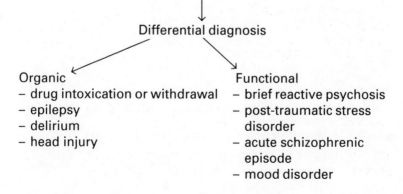

Organic
– drug intoxication or withdrawal
– epilepsy
– delirium
– head injury

Functional
– brief reactive psychosis
– post-traumatic stress disorder
– acute schizophrenic episode
– mood disorder

B.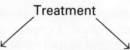

Brief reactive psychosis
– short-term antipsychotics
– supportive psychotherapy
– individual/group/family
   psychotherapy
– antidepressants

Post-traumatic stress disorder
– cognitive therapy
– brief dynamic psychotherapy
– group/family therapy
– short-term antipsychotics

The first step would be to ensure that there are no organic causes of the patient's acute psychotic state, particularly since she was involved in a RTA. The major functional disorders that could present with this clinical picture are outlined in the flow diagram. A brief reactive psychosis (BRP) would follow a significant stressor, with abrupt onset and short duration of acute symptoms (hours to days). The following features, if present, would suggest BRP rather than an acute schizophrenic episode : the presence of affective symptoms, confusion, minimal or no affective blunting, better premorbid adjustment and lack of schizoid personality traits. She has experienced a traumatic episode previously, and therefore is at higher risk of developing BRP. BRP is commoner in adolescents and young adults.

A post-traumatic stress disorder (PTSD) is likely, if her belief that she is being raped does not reach delusional intensity and she appears to be reliving the experience of the rape. It is usual to find that the patients tend to avoid associated stimuli (in this case she could be avoiding going out on her own or relationships with men), persistently re-experience the event in some way and have a heightened awareness of it on the anniversary of the event. There may be evidence of diminished interest in usual activities, sleep disturbance, irritability, poor concentration, high arousal, etc. In this patient's case, the lack of any of these symptoms prior to the accident would not, however, rule out a PTSD, as the stress of the accident could well have precipitated her reliving the experience of her rape.

The treatment of BRP and PTSD is outlined in the flow diagram. In a brief reactive psychosis, the aims of psychotherapy are to encourage the development of coping skills that would help the patient in moments of acute stress and to improve self-esteem and self-confidence. In PTSD, psychotherapy would aim to help the patient overcome denial of the event and avoidance of related stimuli. Relaxation therapy would help her overcome the high level of arousal that is often present. Drugs should only be used in the short term, and antidepressants could be helpful. Follow-up is essential, as her acute psychotic episode in the face of stress could indicate a highly vulnerable personality, or the beginning of a schizophrenic illness.

FURTHER READING

Stephens J H, Shaffer J W, Carpenter W T 1982 Reactive psychosis. Journal of Nervous and Mental Diseases 170(11): 657–663

See also Q21

A53

35-year-old male with Down's syndrome, withdrawn, not eating after recent move

Assessment
– home visit with social worker
– complete history from staff and other sources
– examine patient and surroundings

Patient-related
Functional, e.g.   Organic, e.g.
– adjustment reaction – infections
– depression   – dementia

Environment-related
– unsatisfactory staff
– poor physical
  surroundings

Treat underlying problem

Discuss with staff and
social worker
Inform local authority
Move patient if necessary

The patient will need to be seen at the home, as various factors in the environment could be contributing to his abnormal behaviour. The staff should be seen first, in order to get a clear account of the onset and progression of the patient's altered behaviour and of any precipitating events. A history of his behaviour during previous periods of care should be obtained, if possible, and his notes studied, if available.

It is important to find out where the patient was moved from, the reason for the move and how he has reacted to it. For example, the move may have been necessary due to illness or death of his primary care-giver, and he may be depressed or mourning the loss. He may be having interpersonal problems at the new home. The staff may be finding some aspects of his behaviour or the demands created by him difficult and, if so, one should find out how they are dealing with it. While talking to the staff, one should assess, as far as is practically possible, the physical and social environment at the home, the attitudes of the staff to their work, their workload and the support they are getting from other agencies.

Physical illness could be present and a searching physical evaluation should be done. Disturbed sleep, a change in his ability to take care of himself and to work, unhappiness, anhedonia and irritability would suggest depression. Noticeable intellectual deterioration and behavioural changes could indicate the development of dementia. Carrying out a mental state examination can be difficult if the patient is unable to express his thoughts and feelings and one needs to rely mainly on observed phenomena.

Treatment depends on the nature of the underlying problem, and the primary care team and social services should be appropriately involved at all stages. Suppose, for example, that the problems are a result of the difficulties the patient is having in adjusting to his new surroundings, and the fact that he is missing his previous carers and social circle, i.e. an adjustment disorder. Treatment would involve explaining the move to him, repeatedly if necessary. He should be encouraged to visit his previous home, if possible, and to maintain contact with his friends and relatives. He should be allowed to express his sadness or anger over the move. In his new surroundings, extra efforts should be made to make him feel at home, and the making of new relationships facilitated. The entire process of readjustment can be difficult and prolonged. The patient should be followed-up by his primary team until the problem is resolved, to monitor his progress and to ensure that there is no other problem that could have been missed at the initial assessment. Depression should not be missed as it is eminently treatable. Similarly, if it appears that the patient is developing dementia, he should be thoroughly investigated (psychological testing, CT scan, etc). This is necessary not only to establish a diagnosis of dementia, but also to rule out depression presenting as dementia, which can be particularly difficult to diagnose in patients with Down's syndrome.

FURTHER READING

Fraser W I, Leudar I, Gray J, Campbell I, 1986 Psychiatric and behaviour disturbance in mental handicap. Journal of Mental Deficiency Research 30: 49–57

Reid A H 1982 The psychiatry of mental handicap. Blackwell Scientific, Oxford

Reiss S 1982 Psychopathology and mental retardation. Mental Retardation 20: 128–132

A54

This delusion may be a symptom of a psychotic disorder, such as schizophrenia, or part of a depressive illness. It may also be the manifestation of a monosymptomatic hypochondriacal psychosis, a paranoid state which is more commonly seen in middle-aged or elderly women, though it may occur at a younger age.

Details of the onset and course of her symptoms, response to treatment, and previous diagnosis must be obtained. Her symptoms are likely to be associated with a recurrence of her previous illness, although they could be related to the emergence of a different condition. Predisposing or precipitating factors should be explored in the assessment. These would include: her social situation (e.g. isolation, family problems); financial and work difficulties (e.g. unemployment); accommodation (e.g. inappropriate conditions, hostel); level of support (e.g. family, social services); and stressful experiences (e.g. unwanted pregnancy). The patient's physical condition should be carefully evaluated. In her mental state examination, the severity of her illness should be established, and it is important to ascertain whether she is likely to act on her delusion (e.g. using a vaginal douche to cleanse herself).

Treatment depends on the nature of her illness. Admission may be required, for example, if she is likely to endanger herself or her pregnancy. In the presence of a psychotic or depressive illness, the use of neuroleptics and antidepressants would be indicated. Medication should be administered cautiously in pregnancy, since both neuroleptics and antidepressants pass through the placenta to the foetus. In the first trimester, drugs should be avoided. If absolutely necessary, the smallest effective dose should be used. Divided doses several times a day (to minimise peaking of plasma levels) are better than single daily doses. If the patient's symptoms are part of a severe depressive illness and she is found to be suicidal or not drinking or eating, electroconvulsive therapy should be considered.

If the patient is severely ill, termination of the pregnancy may be indicated on medical grounds. If indicated, her pregnancy can be terminated up to the 24th week. If her pregnancy is continued, liaison with obstetric and midwifery services should be ensured. If possible, the father should be seen. The level of support that the patient needs until delivery and afterwards should be established by the multidisciplinary team.

If the patient's level of functioning and self-care are found to be appropriate, and her condition does not require admission, she can be treated as an outpatient. Counselling, supportive psychotherapy and other psychological treatments (psychodynamic, cognitive, group therapy) may be helpful. A social worker could help the patient to find suitable accommodation and organise her finances. A network involving the general practitioner, health visitor, a community psychiatric nurse and social services should be mobilised. Provisions for perinatal care (e.g. liaison with a mother-and-baby unit) will have to be planned in advance.

FURTHER READING

Appleby L, Fox H, Shaw M, Kumar R 1989 The psychiatrist in the obstetric unit: establishing a liaison service. British Journal of Psychiatry 154: 510–515

Chiu S, McFarlane A H, Dobson N 1990 The treatment of monodelusional psychosis associated with depression. British Journal of Psychiatry 156: 112–115

Munro A 1980 Monosymptomatic hypochondriacal psychosis. British Journal of Hospital Medicine 24: 34–38

A55

This is a middle-aged man who is presenting with symptoms of cognitive impairment, anxiety and depression, associated with abnormal movements of his face and hands. In addition, there is a first-degree relative who was psychiatrically ill.

Abnormal movements and evidence of an incipient dementing process, especially at this patient's age, are likely to be features of Huntington's disease, which is transmitted by a single autosomal dominant gene with 100% penetrance. Diagnosis is based on the positive family history, mental changes and the presence of abnormal movements. In the early stages, Huntington's chorea may be misdiagnosed as other psychiatric or neurological illnesses. Initial manifestations may be those of a functional disorder, such as depression, anxiety or schizophrenia, or may resemble Parkinson's disease, cerebellar disorders, multiple sclerosis or Wilson's disease.

The onset and course of the patient's psychiatric symptoms should be explored with his wife. Emotional disturbance and personality changes may be early signs of the disease. She should be asked about her husband's performance at work and in his daily routine, e.g. his ability to plan and schedule activities. Cognitive deterioration may precede involuntary movements, although symptoms of dementia usually occur after the appearance of abnormal movements. He may appear to have become fidgety and clumsy due to his movements, e.g. flexion and extension of the fingers, facial grimaces, and it is important to know whether these disappear in sleep as is observed in Huntington's disease.

On examination, the patient's gait may be ataxic and the deep tendon reflexes increased, His speech may be dysarthric or irregular, and lurches and jerks noted in his handwriting. He may be unable to copy movements such as furrowing the brow or blowing out the cheeks. On mental state examination, symptoms of depression and anxiety may be elicited. Delusions and hallucinations may occur. In the assessment of his cognitive functions, deficits in attention and spatial judgement may be found. In Huntington's disease, however, memory is relatively spared, with disorientation in time and space being noted only at late stages. Moreover, dysphasia, dyslexia and agnosia are seldom observed.

It is essential that details of his father's history are obtained along with information about other siblings and relatives. Further investigations may include an EEG and a brain CT scan. In the early stages, the EEG shows low-voltage fast activity. Characteristically, there is an almost complete loss of alpha rhythm. At later stages, a diffuse, slow activity is observed. Typical findings in CT scan include dilated ventricles, cortical atrophy and atrophy of caudate nuclei.

The impact of the diagnosis for the patient and his family must be carefully handled. This includes support and advice for aspects such as work, morale and long-term family decisions, and genetic counselling and testing (DNA analysis) for the relatives. Help from social services will be important in order to provide continuing care. Depressive or psychotic episodes may occur and should be treated accordingly. Medication with neuroleptics can help to control choreiform movements.

FURTHER READING

Bolt J M W 1970 Huntington's chorea in the West of Scotland. British Journal of Psychiatry 116: 259–270

Chase T N, Wexler N S, Barbeau A (eds) 1979 Huntington's disease. Advances in neurology, Vol. 23. Raven Press, New York

Dewhurst K, Oliver J E, McKnight A L 1970 Socio-psychiatric consequences of Huntington's disease. British Journal of Psychiatry 116: 255–258

Martindale B 1987 Huntington's chorea: some psychodynamics seen in those at risk and in the responses of the helping professions. British Journal of Psychiatry 150: 319–323

A56

This is a woman who has bipolar affective disorder and has had two episodes of hypomania and one of depression, before treatment was initiated at the age of 39. She has responded well to treatment with lithium, despite the fact that 30–50% of patients are said not to respond to this treatment.

The first step would be to find out the details of her previous episodes of illness. Information should be obtained from her medical notes and from her general practitioner. The details of her lithium treatment, including her compliance with treatment and whether she had adequate blood levels, should be obtained. The next step would be to find out why she wants to stop her treatment. Is she just tired of taking tablets everyday? Does she want to have a child? Is she experiencing any side-effects, such as renal or thyroid dysfunction? Many patients discontinue their treatment because of weight gain. The decision to discontinue the lithium carbonate will be influenced by these reasons as well as the risk of relapse following discontinuation of treatment. Her previous history shows that she was considered at risk of relapse without this form of medication, and this should be discussed with her in considerable detail. All the consequences of relapse need to be made clear – disruption to her life, her family, her work and the emotional and economic cost. This is usually done by pointing out her current stable condition compared with her previous difficulties. If she has any plans, for example changing her job or going abroad, it should be pointed out to her that periods of turbulence might provoke relapse.

If she wishes to discontinue the medication because of side-effects, she needs careful physical examination as well as investigation of her thyroid and renal function. Thyroid dysfunction is not an absolute contraindication to the use of lithium. Hypothyroidism may be controlled by the concomitant prescription of small doses of thyroxine (0.05–0.2 mg) daily. Renal or cardiovascular dysfunction, similarly, are relative contraindications to the use of lithium carbonate. She may be advised to take carbamazepine instead of lithium carbonate in these circumstances. Weight gain may be controlled by dietary advice. Dermatological side-effects, such as psoriasis, may be more difficult to manage and do remit when the lithium is discontinued.

Should the patient wish not to have any medication, she should be advised to follow a programme of very gradual withdrawal, with careful monitoring of her mental state over a long period because of the serious risk of relapse.

FURTHER READING

Janicek P G, O'Connor E 1990 Major affective disorders: issues involving recovery and recurrence. Current Opinion in Psychiatry 3: 48–53

Prien R F, Kupfer D J, Mansky P A 1984 Drug therapy in the prevention of recurrences in unipolar and bipolar affective disorders. Archives of General Psychiatry 41: 1096–1104

Silverstone T, Romans–Clarkson S 1989 Bipolar affective disorders, causes and prevention of relapse. British Journal of Psychiatry 154: 321–335

A57

The problem is that of a 69-year-old woman with a long psychiatric history who is very disturbed and has absconded before the social workers could give an opinion.

The immediate problem is that an elderly woman thought to be at risk, or who might put other people at risk, is unsupervised in the community. The immediate response should be to alert all relevant people about her disappearance. Although she is not under a section, it would still be important to report her to the police as a missing person. Her family and friends should be informed, and all her old haunts checked as far as possible.

If the woman is found by the police and she is willing to come to hospital, they may bring her directly to hospital. If she is unwilling to be taken to the hospital, they may use Section 136 of the Mental Health Act to hold her in a place of safety whilst the necessary assessments are carried out. The police will usually endeavour to bring the person directly to the hospital (as the place of safety) on S136 for these assessments.

If the woman is found by family or friends, the nearest relative can make the application for compulsory admission. If the family are not willing or able to make the application, an emergency social work assessment should be requested. The medical recommendations can be used for 14 days after completion.

The nursing home should be asked to keep her place until she is found and reassessed, and a decision made as to whether she is able to return there or whether more sheltered or intensive care is required.

A58

45-year-old barrister, four days post-RTA, disturbed and uncontrollable

Direct consequence of RTA, e.g.
- head injury
- infection
- electrolyte imbalance

Totally unrelated to RTA, e.g. pre-existing functional illness

Precipitated by RTA or its treatment, e.g.:
- anaesthetic complications
- alcohol/drug withdrawal

In order to advise on management, it is important to establish as far as possible the cause of the disturbed behaviour. Some of this can be ascertained before seeing the patient, by discussion with the ward staff and examination of the case notes. Additional information should be sought from an informant who knows the patient well, and by a phone call to his general practitioner.

Details of the patient's past psychiatric history would help to exclude certain possibilities, such as pre-existing functional illness. The details of the RTA – whether he sustained a head injury or not – and the treatment thereafter, e.g. administration of a general anaesthetic, should be ascertained.

Given the onset of the problems four days post-RTA, it is highly likely that the problem is related to alcohol withdrawal. In order to establish the diagnosis, it would be useful to ascertain:

- previous history of excessive drinking and/or drink related problems
- whether alcohol was implicated in the RTA
- evidence of chronic alcohol use on physical examination, e.g. stigmata of chronic liver damage
- evidence of alcohol abuse in laboratory tests, such as erythrocyte mean cell volume and gamma glutamyl transferase.

Further assessment of the patient would seek to clarify gaps in the history as well as examination of the mental state.

In delirium tremens (DTs) there is usually rapidly changing mental state, with agitation, restlessness, fearfulness and shouting. This is accompanied by vivid visual hallucinations (sometimes other hallucinations), clouding of consciousness, disorientation in time and place and impairment of recent memory. There is gross tremor of the hands, and the patient may pick at imaginary objects on the bedclothes. The patient will usually display autonomic disturbances, such as sweating, tachycardia, high blood pressure, dilatation of pupils and fever. He is also likely to be dehydrated.

Untreated delirium tremens has a substantial mortality (5%), so treatment is of some urgency. Treatment includes nursing in a quiet, well-lit room, rehydration, sedation with benzodiazepines, and vitamins.

For a more detailed discussion of treatment. See Q45

FURTHER READING

Chick J 1989 Delirium tremens. British Medical Journal 1298: 3

Redfern T R, Rees D, Owen R 1988 The impact of alcohol ingestion on the orthopaedic and accident service. Alcohol 23: 415–420

Royal College of Psychiatrists 1986 Alcohol, our favourite drug: a new report of a special committee. Tavistock, London

A59

The first step is to establish what has happened in the last two weeks. There may have been considerable change in the patient's condition in this time. Life events may have occurred that have caused the patient to become depressed and hence suicidal. It is also possible that the patient did have a formal psychiatric disorder that was undetected during his recent admission.

A decision should then be made as to whether the patient should be seen as an emergency, or whether he should be seen at a regular outpatient clinic or possibly referred to some non-psychiatric agency for help with his difficulties. The decision to see him immediately would be taken if he is thought to have developed some psychiatric problems, or if he is thought to be a serious suicide risk. There would be increased risk of deliberate self-harm if he has attempted suicide in the past, if he is from social class 4 or 5, if he is separated or divorced, if he is a habitual drug user or if he has been drinking, especially recently. If his history suggests that he makes frequent suicidal threats in order to see a psychiatrist or to get admission to hospital, this behaviour should not be reinforced by offering an immediate appointment or hospital admission.

When the patient is seen, a very detailed assessment should be carried out. It is important to try to understand why the patient has been threatening to kill himself, what the degree of intent is – i.e. whether he remains a serious suicide risk – and what problems confront him. Even if he has no formal psychiatric disorder, it is necessary to establish what form of help would be appropriate. He may benefit from brief problem-oriented treatment. The aim would be to help the patient to separate out his problems and find ways of sorting out each one. The five stages of brief problem-oriented therapy are assessment of the immediate problem, help with sorting out that particular crisis, help with ways of coping with subsequent crises without resorting to threats of suicide, termination of the treatment and follow-up.

FURTHER READING

Hawton K, Catalan J 1987 Attempted suicide. A practical guide to its nature and management, 2nd ed. Oxford Medical Publications, Oxford

A60

A.   Acute behavioural disturbance in a male homosexual patient on a medical ward, possibly HIV-related

↓

Obtain all medical and nursing details
Complete psychiatric and cognitive assessment

↓

Differential diagnosis

Major depression
Adjustment disorder
Pathological anxiety/phobia

Delirium
Dementia
Psychosis

(All of the above could be secondary to or unrelated to, physical complications of HIV infection, e.g. severe infections, neoplasia, toxic or metabolic abnormalities, encephalopathy.)

B. Treatment
– immediate sedation if required
– transfer to psychiatric ward if unmanageable
– treat underlying condition
– support staff
– help staff reassure and deal with other patients
– HIV testing and counselling at appropriate time with consent

There are three aspects to this clinical problem:

1. carrying out a psychiatric assessment and dealing with the immediate problem of the patient's disturbed behaviour
2. dealing with HIV-testing refusal
3. helping the staff on the ward deal with their anxiety and with the other patients.

1. While discussing the patient with the referring team, it is important to find whether the medical team thinks he is likely to have clinical HIV disease, and if there could be other physical or iatrogenic reasons for his depression. During this discussion, it should also be possible to assess whether the staff are likely to need any practical help or support.

In the assessment, one should look specifically for evidence of an acute confusional state, focal or global cognitive impairment, depression, suicidal ideation, pathological anxiety, phobias, and psychotic features. At this stage, one will be in a position to say whether the patient is mentally ill or not, and consider whether the illness is likely to be related to HIV infection. Further treatment depends on the nature of the problem.

Given the disturbed state of the patient, it may not be possible to proceed in the logical manner described. The first decision that may need to be taken is that of sedation to calm him down. This can be achieved with an antipsychotic (chlorpromazine, haloperidol) and/or a benzodiazepine (diazepam), provided his disturbed behaviour is not a consequence of an acute organic state. If it is more appropriate to nurse him on a psychiatric ward, a transfer should be organised. If he is unwilling to be admitted or treated, then it would be appropriate to consider a compulsory admission under the Mental Health Act, provided his disturbed behaviour is thought to be related to an underlying psychiatric illness. Pending further examination and investigations, the patient should be treated as HIV-positive, and appropriate precautions and isolation procedures should be implemented.

2. The second part of the question deals with the problem of HIV test refusal. In this instance, knowing the HIV status of the patient will allow the staff to (1) use appropriate precautions and isolate him if his behaviour necessitates it and (2) give him the appropriate treatment. The first can be done *without* a positive test result, if it is felt that the risk of infection is significant. If the patient is mentally ill, and his refusal is a result of this, then the first priority is to treat his mental illness. His decision may change after successful treatment. HIV testing cannot be carried out under any section of the Mental Health Act without consent of the patient, *unless* the psychiatric condition is thought to be a direct result of HIV infection, and testing forms part of the management of the psychiatric disorder. Even in such an instance, the decision to test should not be taken without involving the team, getting a second psychiatric and/or other expert opinion, and consulting the Department of Health, the General Medical Council and a relevant medical defence society. If the patient is mentally well and refuses testing, one cannot carry out the test. In this situation, general education about the illness and pre-test counselling may change a patient's mind, and should be tried if he agrees.

3. The other patients on the ward, and the staff are clearly worried about the possibility of infection. It may be necessary to use appropriate disinfecting methods (wash with soap and water, encourage bleeding from wounds, report to medical officer), and wash and disinfect contaminated areas of the ward with hypochlorite or glutaraldehyde. The patient should be isolated if his disturbed behaviour continues. The other patients should be reassured, and appropriately educated by the staff. It would be useful to get a health and safety official or AIDS counsellor to talk to the patients and staff about their concerns. The psychiatrist can help develop staff support facilities if these are lacking.

FURTHER READING

Advisory Committee on Dangerous Pathogens 1990 HIV – the causative agent of AIDS and related conditions, 2nd revision of guidelines. HMSO, London

Catalan J, Riccio M, Thompson C, 1989 HIV disease and psychiatric practice. Psychiatric Bulletin 13 : 316–322

Departments of Health 1990 Guidance for clinical health care workers: protection against infection with HIV and hepatitis viruses. HMSO, London

Evans D L, Perkins D O 1990 The clinical psychiatry of AIDS. Current Opinion in Psychiatry 3: 96–102

General Medical Council 1988 HIV infection and AIDS: the ethical considerations. General Medical Council, London

See also Q6 and Q14.

Recommended Texts

American Psychiatric Association, 1987 Diagnostic and statistical manual of mental disorders, 3rd edn, revised. American Psychiatric Association, Washington D C

Bebbington P E, Hill P 1985 Manual of clinical psychiatry. Blackwell Scientific, Oxford

Bluglass R S 1983 A guide to the Mental Health Act 1983. Churchill Livingstone, Edinburgh

Bluglass R, Bowden P (eds) 1990 Principles and practice of forensic psychiatry. Churchill Livingstone, Edinburgh

Department of Health and Welsh Office 1990 Code of practice: Mental Health Act 1983. HMSO, London

Department of Health and Social Security 1983 The Mental Health Act. HMSO, London

Gelder M, Gath D, Mayou R 1989 Oxford textbook of psychiatry. Oxford University Press, Oxford

Graham P 1986 Child psychiatry: a developmental approach. Oxford University Press, Oxford

Hersov L, Rutter M 1985 Child psychiatry: modern approaches, 2nd edn. Blackwell Scientific, Oxford

Hill P, Murray R, Thorley A (eds) 1986 Essentials of post-graduate psychiatry. Grune and Stratton, New York

Kaplan H I, Sadock B J (eds) 1987 Comprehensive textbook of psychiatry, 4th edn, Williams and Wilkins, Baltimore

Kendell R E, Zealley A K (eds) 1989 Companion to psychiatric studies. Churchill Livingstone, Edinburgh

Lishman W A 1987 Organic psychiatry; the psychological consequences of cerebral disorder, 2nd edn. Blackwell Scientific, Oxford

Marks I M 1987 Fears, phobias and rituals. Oxford University Press, New York

McGuffin P, Shanks M F, Hodgson M F (eds) 1984 The scientific principles of psychopathology. Grune and Stratton, New York

Royal College of Psychiatrists 1986 Alcohol, our favourite drug: a new report of a special committee. Tavistock, London

Shepherd M (general editor) 1983 Handbook of psychiatry. Cambridge University Press, Cambridge
   Vol. 1   Shepherd M, Zangwill O L General psychopathology.
   Vol. 2   Lader M H Mental disorder and somatic illness.
   Vol. 3   Wing J K, Wing L Psychoses of uncertain aetiology.
   Vol. 4   Russel G F M, Hersov L A The neuroses and personality disorders
   Vol. 5   Shepherd M The scientific foundations of psychiatry.

World Health Organization 1977 International Classification of Diseases, revision 9. WHO, Geneva

Index

Questions are given in ordinary type and answers in **bold**.